T0215328

Qualitative Research Methodologies for Occupational Science and Therapy

The push for evidence-based practice has increased the demand for high-quality occupational science and occupational therapy research from conceptualization of the study to publication. This invaluable collection explores how to produce rigorous qualitative research by presenting and discussing a range of methodologies and methods that can be used in the fields of occupational science and therapy.

Each chapter, written by an experienced researcher in the relevant methodology, includes examples of research, foundational knowledge and therapeutic applications. Including new and cutting-edge methodologies, the book covers:

Qualitative Descriptive
Grounded Theory
Phenomenology
Narrative
Ethnography
Action Research
Case Study
Critical Discourse Analysis
Visual Methodologies
Meta-synthesis
Appreciative Inquiry
Critical Theory and Philosophy

Designed for occupational science and occupational therapy researchers, this book develops the reader's ability to produce and critique high-quality qualitative research that is epistemologically sound and rigorous.

Shoba Nayar is a Senior Lecturer in the postgraduate public health program at the School of Public Health and Psychosocial Studies, and Associate Director of the Centre for Migrant and Refugee Research, Auckland University of Technology, New Zealand. Shoba is the President of the Association of the Journal of Occupational Science and an associate editor for the *Journal of Occupational Science*.

Mandy Stanley is a Senior Lecturer in the occupational therapy program at the School of Health Science and member of the International Center for Allied Health Evidence, University of South Australia, Australia. Mandy is the President of the Australasian Society of Occupational Scientists and an associate editor for the *Journal of Occupational Science*.

Qualitative Research Methodologies for Occupational Science and Therapy

Edited by Shoba Nayar and Mandy Stanley

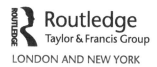

Routledge
Taylor & Francis Group

LONDON AND NEW YORK

First published 2015 by Routledge

2 Park Square, Milton Park, Abingdon, Oxon OX14 4RN
711 Third Avenue, New York, NY 10017, USA

Routledge is an imprint of the Taylor & Francis Group, an informa business

First issued in paperback 2016

British Library Cataloguing-in-Publication Data
A catalogue record for this book is available from the British Library

Library of Congress Cataloging-in-Publication Data
Qualitative research methodologies for occupational science and therapy/
edited by Shoba Nayar and Mandy Stanley.
p.;cm.
Includes bibliographical references.
I. Nayar, Shoba, editor. II. Stanley, Mandy, Dr., editor.
[DNLM: 1. Occupational Medicine. 2. Research Design. 3. Occupational
Therapy. 4. Qualitative Research. WA 20.5]
RM735
615.8′515—dc23
2014018265

ISBN: 978-0-415-82867-3 (hbk)
ISBN: 978-1-138-28350-3 (pbk)

Typeset in Times New Roman
by Swales & Willis Ltd, Exeter, Devon, UK

To Zach, Cleo and Sii Tao; and Jeremy, Val and Krish.
With love and thanks . . .

Contents

Illustrations

Figures

Tables

Boxes

Editor biographies

Shoba Nayar, PhD

Associate Director, Centre for Migrant and Refugee Research, and Senior Lecturer, Department of Public Health, School of Public Health and Psychosocial Studies, Faculty of Health & Environmental Sciences, AUT University, Auckland, New Zealand.

My first international journey occurred at the age of 14 months when I emigrated with my family from England to New Zealand. Since that time I have been a regular international traveler, living in various parts of the world. These experiences, and my practice as an occupational therapist and occupational scientist, have ignited my passion as a qualitative researcher in understanding how refugee and Asian immigrant communities experience and manage issues of transition and well-being.

Mandy Stanley, PhD

Senior Lecturer, Occupational Therapy Program, International Centre for Allied Health Evidence, School of Health Sciences, University of South Australia, Adelaide, Australia.

Two pivotal moments in my academic career have influenced the researcher that I am today. First, working with Prof. Ann Wilcock at the time that she launched the *Journal of Occupational Science*, and second, meeting with the late Prof. Gary Kielhofner who guided me in the direction of choosing a qualitative research methodology for my doctoral studies. My contribution to this book would not have come about without those moments and my enthusiasm for the occupational therapy profession.

Contributors

Sissel Alsaker, PhD Associate Professor, Department of Nursing, Sör-Tröndelag University College, Trondheim, Norway

Eric Asaba, PhD Associate Professor, Division of Occupational Therapy, Department of Neurobiology, Care Sciences and Society, Karolinska Institutet, Solna, Sweden

Silke Dennhardt, PhD Research Associate and Research Coordinator, Centre for Education Research & Innovation, Schulich School of Medicine & Dentistry, University of Western Onatrio, London, ON, Canada

Danika Galvin, BHthSc(OT) PhD Candidate, Charles Sturt University, Albury, Australia

Clare Hocking, PhD Professor, Department of Occupational Science and Therapy, Auckland University of Technology, Auckland, New Zealand

Suzanne Huot, PhD Assistant Professor, School of Occupational Therapy, University of Western Ontario, London, ON, Canada

Margaret Jones, MHSc Lecturer, Department of Occupational Science and Therapy, Auckland University of Technology, Auckland, New Zealand

Staffan Josephsson, PhD Professor, Division of Occupational Therapy, Department of Neurobiology, Care Sciences and Society, Karolinska Institutet, Solna, Sweden

Debbie Laliberte Rudman, PhD Associate Professor, School of Occupational Therapy and Graduate Program in Health and Rehabilitation Sciences, Faculty of Health Sciences, University of Western Ontario, London, ON, Canada

Jenni Mace, MSc H&SS Senior Lecturer, Department of Occupational Science and Therapy, Auckland University of Technology, Auckland, New Zealand

Margarita Mondaca, MSc OT Lecturer, Division of Occupational Therapy, Department of Neurobiology, Care Sciences and Society, Karolinska Institutet, Solna, Sweden

Carolyn Murray, MOT PhD Candidate Lecturer, Occupational Therapy Program, International Centre of Allied Health Evidence, School of Health Sciences, University of South Australia, Adelaide, Australia

Shoba Nayar, PhD Associate Director, Centre for Migrant and Refugee Research, Auckland University of Technology, Auckland, New Zealand

Melissa Park, PhD Assistant Professor, School of Physical & Occupational Therapy, Faculty of Medicine, McGill University, Montréal, QC, Canada

Ben Sellar, PhD Lecturer, Department of Occupational Therapy, University of South Australia, Adelaide, Australia

Mandy Stanley, PhD Senior Lecturer, Occupational Therapy Program, International Centre for Allied Health Evidence, School of Health Sciences, University of South Australia, Adelaide, Australia

Marilyn Waring, PhD Professor of Public Policy, Institute of Public Policy, Auckland University of Technology, Auckland, New Zealand

Clare Wilding, PhD Director, Knowledge Moves, Beechworth, Australia Adjunct Senior Lecturer, School of Community Health, Charles Sturt University, Albury, Australia

Valerie Wright-St Clair, PhD Associate Professor, Department of Occupational Science and Therapy, School of Rehabilitation and Occupation Studies, Faculty of Health & Environmental Sciences, Auckland University of Technology, Auckland, New Zealand

Acknowledgments

Our thanks to Valerie Wright-St Clair for being a critical friend and to Shoshannah Williams for her research skills. We thank the team at Routledge for their support throughout the process. We also acknowledge the support of our respective universities: Auckland University of Technology and University of South Australia. Finally, we thank our colleagues who so willingly gave their time and expertise as contributing authors.

1 Beginning conversations

Shoba Nayar and Mandy Stanley

Our story

The idea for this book came from a number of conversations that we have had over time. At various points over the past few years, when we came together from our homes in Australia and Aotearoa New Zealand at conferences or meetings, we would have a conversation about qualitative research. We often lamented that the quality of some of the published qualitative research within occupational science and occupational therapy was not what it could and should be. The publishing of studies of low methodological quality raised particular areas of concern.

First, we questioned whether the studies demonstrated the appropriate level of respect for participants who volunteer time and allow researchers access to aspects of their personal lives. Such studies, we believe, do not do justice to those volunteers and may be a poor reflection on the occupational science discipline or the occupational therapy profession. Second, with the growing demand for evidence-based practice, we were concerned about the quality of evidence. Already, researchers and practitioners who subscribe to a hierarchy of evidence based on understanding causation do not rate qualitative research highly; and it certainly will not be well regarded if it is not quality work. But further, if the profession at large wants occupational therapy practice to be based on research evidence, then it must be quality evidence to inform practice. If practitioners are drawing on published studies that are of low quality, then it will not be the best evidence for quality occupational therapy practice and good outcomes for clients.

The third concern centered on how the profession's body of knowledge would be judged by other researchers and practitioners, based on their reading of the published literature if the quality is low. To be taken seriously by service funders and other professions, occupational science and occupational therapy researchers must show that they can produce and disseminate quality studies. Given our shared concerns we came to the decision that instead of lamenting the situation, we should do something more positive and make an active contribution to remedying the situation as we perceive it.

We are both occupational scientists and occupational therapists, as well as qualitative researchers with experience as university academics. We use qualitative approaches within our own work and in our supervision of research students, and we have experience teaching qualitative methodologies. We review for a number of occupational therapy and health-related journals and are associate editors for the *Journal of Occupational Science*. But rather than laying out our curriculum vitae at this point, we prefer to convey our passion in relation to both occupational science and occupational therapy and qualitative research.

Our shared interests and experience, and commitment to positive contributions, led us to writing a paper together for an occupational therapy audience about improving the quality of qualitative research. While writing that paper, we came to the realization that our ideas could be expanded and perhaps it would make a better book than a journal article. So once we finished the paper we worked on the book proposal. While working on the proposal we facilitated a workshop at a New Zealand Association Occupational Therapy national conference, which was based on our manuscript and some of our emerging ideas. We had a positive response to that workshop, from both novice and experienced researchers, which reinforced to us the need for this book. In developing the book proposal we canvassed existing texts which supported our claim, as it appeared that this was the first time a methodological text was being mooted that brought together occupational science and occupational therapy and that had a specific methodological focus on researching occupation. Occupational science and occupational therapy have reached a stage of maturity in discipline and professional growth warranting the publication of occupation-focused research texts. Despite the explicit focus on occupational science and occupational therapy, researchers from other disciplines may well find something useful and relevant in this book.

Without making claims to know it all, we have set out to create a text that might provide some guidance to students and novice researchers or to experienced researchers who want to extend their knowledge and skills into methodologies less familiar to them. We offer that guidance with humility and recognize our limitations, so it is not the definitive text, rather we put it forward as a contribution. Our intent right from the beginning was to have a strong international flavor. Thus, a key feature of this book is the inclusion of chapter contributions from leading occupational science and occupational therapy researchers from across the globe, bringing variety, depth, and breadth.

Focus of the book

Qualitative research approaches have been used in both occupational science and occupational therapy research for some time. So what do we mean when we the use term qualitative research? Nkwi, Nyamongo and Ryan (2001) stated that "Qualitative research involves any research that uses data that do not indicate ordinal values" (p. 1). This is deliberately a broad and all-encompassing definition. While still maintaining the breadth, Denzin and Lincoln (2005) offered a somewhat more refined definition, "Qualitative researchers study things in their natural settings, attempting to make sense of, or to interpret, phenomena in terms of the meanings people bring to them" (p. 3). In this book, and in our practice, we conceptualize qualitative research as a process of conversation either with oneself and/or with others, be they individuals or groups or dialoguing with texts.

As conversations vary, so too do different approaches within qualitative research. Some are descriptive, some are more in-depth, some are designed with a specific purpose to understand or get behind a topic and so on. Essentially, we believe, as with any good conversation, qualitative research is about authentic engagement with the context within which one is situated, for the purpose of advancing understandings in the topic of interest. To fully develop those understandings, the conversation requires thought and planning, as well as a commitment to ensuring a rigorous process, which is not without its challenges. Thus, in choosing to undertake qualitative research, one should not underestimate the demand or the effort required to do it well.

To produce rigorous qualitative research, that is credible both within academic scholarship and the wider community of health professionals, occupational scientists and occupational therapists need to have a solid understanding of the match between topic, question, methodology, and methods. Without these understandings translated into good research practice, there is a risk that the discipline and profession fail to produce quality evidence that can be taken seriously and used judiciously by those who hold and sit outside of an occupational perspective. Hence, the purpose of this book is to explore a range of qualitative research methodologies and related methods that can be used in the fields of occupational science and therapy.

At this point, it is important to acknowledge that while the focus of this text is very clearly on qualitative research, it is not to say that we do not value quantitative research. In our view, approaches to research form a continuum with quantitative and qualitative at opposite ends and mixed methodology claiming middle ground. We certainly do not want to perpetuate any debates of quantitative versus qualitative work as each has its own value and purpose. For us it is about choosing the right approach for the research question. Currently, the questions in occupational science and occupational therapy that energize us and call to be answered are best served by a qualitative methodology.

In the occupational therapy practice arena, there is a strong push from funders and clients to have practice that is evidence based. Evidence-based practice, developed out of evidence-based medicine, is defined as practice that is informed by a combination of client preference, practitioner expertise, and the research evidence (Sackett, Strauss, Richardson, Rosenberg, & Haynes, 2000). In our experience that definition, which emphasizes the combination of the three areas, is played out with the research evidence trumping practitioner experience and expertise. Furthermore the research evidence is then classified into a hierarchy by eminent governing bodies of research such as the National Institute of Health (United States) and National Health and Medical Research Council (Australia). In those evidence hierarchies, qualitative research ranks quite low in the hierarchy.

When it comes to single studies examining questions about effectiveness of interventions, randomized controlled trials, often considered to be the gold standard, will provide the best research evidence. There has been a concerted push for robust trials and systematic reviews; however, in many areas of occupational therapy, evidence from randomized controlled trials just does not exist. Much of what occupational therapists do in practice is difficult to reduce to discrete variables that can be measured and controlled, in large part due to the complexity of occupational engagement, the diversity of individuals and environments, and the nature of the relationship between the occupational therapist and the client.

Other authors have critiqued the philosophical fit between occupational therapy and evidence-based practice (Gustafson, Molineux, & Bennet, 2014), but it would be remiss of us not to address the issue in this text. The need for evidence for practice is not being questioned; what we are questioning is the place of qualitative research within that evidence. For questions related to the client's view of a particular intervention, use of a qualitative methodology will provide the best research evidence. Qualitative research methodologies can account for the complexity of occupational engagement situated in context. As such, Tomlin and Borgetto (2011) have proposed an alternative hierarchy of evidence which is a three-dimensional pyramid with three sides and a base. One of the sides is the hierarchy of qualitative evidence with qualitative studies utilizing one source of data at the lowest rank on the hierarchy and meta-syntheses which combine a number of related qualitative studies at the top. The authors acknowledge that there are some limitations to their proposed model; however, it is worthy of consideration.

As a contribution to building research capacity, to generate the research evidence for occupational therapy, we see this book as a first stop for occupational scientists or occupational therapists interested in undertaking qualitative research with an explicit occupational focus, but do not believe that it is the only stop. Within the chapters, authors have directed readers to other quality resources for more in-depth consideration of the chosen methodology. We encourage readers to explore these resources and further readings, while knowing they can always return to this text that it is 'grounded in occupation'.

The intended audience is primarily graduate students in the fields of occupational science and occupational therapy with a basic understanding of qualitative research approaches; however, graduate students and researchers from other health disciplines may also benefit.

A key feature of this book is the inclusion of chapters that thus far have not been considered in other occupational therapy texts. These chapters address new and cutting edge research methodologies including meta-synthesis, visual methodologies, and critical theory.

The chapters

Each chapter is written by an occupational scientist/therapist who has experience in the particular methodological approach. Throughout the chapters, examples of research pertaining to occupation, in terms of both foundational knowledge (occupational science) and therapeutic applications (occupational therapy), are used to showcase the application of the methodological approach. The aim is to develop the reader's ability to produce high-quality qualitative research that is epistemologically sound and rigorous and to be a skilled critical reader of qualitative research.

Having introduced ourselves as editors, sharing the story of how we came to be writing this book and declaring our intent, we turn in Chapter 2 to consider a brief history of qualitative research within occupational science and occupational therapy and to set forth some shared understandings that underpin the qualitative methodologies explicated in the following chapters.

The specific methodology chapters begin with Chapter 3 on qualitative descriptive. Mandy Stanley draws on her experience of conducting research with a team to explore older Australians' perspectives on loneliness, while in Chapter 4, Shoba Nayar utilizes her work related to Indian immigrant women settling in New Zealand to reveal the process of grounded theory methodology.

Chapter 5 on phenomenology has been written by New Zealand researcher Valerie Wright-St Clair. In this chapter, Valerie relates her experience of becoming a phenomenologist and the value of the methodology in revealing the ordinary in the everyday. Multiple examples from her reflective journal and data are used to explicate the art of phenomenology.

Researchers from Sweden and Norway, Staffan Josephsson and Sissel Alsaker, respond to the call for an elaborated and sensitive qualitative inquiry within occupational science and occupational therapy through their exploration of narrative methodology and argue that narrative moves beyond solely 'words'. Next we travel to Canada, where Suzanne Huot captures the essence of ethnography in Chapter 7 through her personal descriptions of the Francophone community in Canada. Suzanne's experience is a powerful reminder of how qualitative research can be a changing experience for both researchers and participants. Noteworthy here is her innovate use of occupational mapping as a data collection approach.

Australian researchers Clare Wilding and Danika Galvin draw on two different action research studies in Chapter 8 to demonstrate the transformative power of action research methodology for studying phenomena in context and embedding occupational science concepts into occupational science practice. In Chapter 9, New Zealand researchers Margaret Jones and Clare Hocking explicate case study methodology and demonstrate the thought and planning that is required in order to produce quality case study research. Their chapter highlights the strength of qualitative research in studying the complexity of occupational engagement, and they use a unique multilayered approach to analyze data both literally and figuratively.

Chapters 10 and 11 are brought to us by a group of international researchers from Canada, Sweden, and Germany. Chapter 10 draws on two Canadian studies by Debbie Laliberte Rudman and Silke Denhardt to introduce readers to critical discourse as a qualitative methodology that uses analysis of texts to address issues of power. Power is also forefronted in Chapter 11 through a visual medium as Eric Asaba, Debbie Laliberte Rudman, Margarita Mondaca, and Melissa Park introduce us to the potential of photovoice as an emerging methodology used in two Swedish and Canadian studies.

Chapter 12 is an insightful discussion of the process of undertaking a meta-synthesis. Australian researchers Carolyn Murray and Mandy Stanley tackle some of the issues of using this methodology in a field where there is sometimes very limited literature and provide a useful framework for undertaking this form of research.

In Chapter 13 New Zealand researcher Jenni Mace and her supervisors Clare Hocking and Marilyn Waring focus on the substantive area of homelessness and the benefit of appreciative inquiry in drawing from a strength-based approach to facilitate possibilities for new futures. In drawing the chapters on specific methodologies to a close, Australian researcher Ben Sellar challenges the reader to use critical theory as a methodology for questioning the construction of power and knowledge in relation to occupation.

In the final chapter we present a group discussion between selected contributing authors regarding what they see as the challenges and strengths of qualitative methodologies, as well as drawing from their own experiences to offer advice to those undertaking research using qualitative methodologies for the first time in their career.

How to navigate the book

The order in which the chapters are presented is deliberate. We start with approaches within an interpretive paradigm (aiming to deepen understandings) before moving to approaches within a critical paradigm (intentionally aimed at making change) before moving to a postmodern paradigm (aiming to celebrate the diversity of life). As is noted within each chapter, there is not one right way to go about applying the research methodology. In reality, it is much more nuanced and researchers can choose from variations within a methodology and from a range of methods. Each author offers one particular slant on a methodology in which there are multiple variations. It is not possible to cover every variation and the purpose here is not to write another *SAGE Handbook of Qualitative Research* (Denzin & Lincoln, 2005).

Each chapter has a similar structure with some variations reflecting the author style and methodology. Beginning with an introduction to the methodology and epistemology, each chapter discusses what the methodology aims to do and suitable topics/questions that might be asked. This leads on to the selection of the particular research methods including recruitment and sampling, data collection and analysis. Throughout, authors draw on their own work to provide examples of the different methods in play. Following the methods, there is a section on ensuring rigor within a study and issues of ethics particular to the chosen methodology. Next, authors offer a set of questions to ask when critiquing studies using the methodology before providing examples of how the given form of qualitative research contributes to occupational science and occupational therapy. The chapter concludes with the authors' personal reflections on their fit/choice of the methodology. At the end of each chapter further resources in the form of additional readings and websites to quality sources are offered to readers to extend their knowledge and skills.

Readers have the choice of beginning with Chapter 1 and reading through to the final chapter, or dipping in and out of chapters as needed. The consistent framework in each chapter enables the reader to readily locate the material they are interested in.

Having begun the conversation about qualitative research here in Chapter 1, we turn next to Chapter 2 to continue our discussion. In particular, our discussion here includes a potted history of qualitative research in occupational science and occupational therapy and a closer examination of key issues to consider related to qualitative research, including, reflexivity, differentiating between epistemology, methodology and methods, and a consideration of the research context. We hope you will enjoy the unfolding conversations.

Happy reading.

References

Denzin, N., & Lincoln, Y. (Eds.). (2005). *Handbook of qualitative research* (3rd ed.). Thousand Oaks, CA: Sage.

Gustafson, L., Molineux, M., & Bennet, S. (2014). Contemporary occupational therapy practice: The challenges of being evidence based and philosophically congruent. *Australian Occupational Therapy Journal, 61*(1), 121–123. doi:10.1111/1441–1630. 12110.

Nkwi, P., Nyamongo, I., & Ryan, G. (2001). *Field research into socio-cultural issues: Methodological guidelines.* Cameroon, Africa: International Center for Applied Social Sciences Research and Training/UNFPA.

Sackett, D. L., Strauss, S. E., Richardson, W. S., Rosenberg, W., & Haynes, R. B. (2000). *Evidence-based medicine: How to practice and teach EBM* (2nd ed.). Edinburgh, Scotland: Churchill Livingstone.

Tomlin, G., & Borgetto, B. (2011). Research pyramid: A new evidence-based practice model for occupational therapy. *American Journal of Occupational Therapy, 65*, 189–196. doi:10.5014/ajot.2011.000828.

2 Deepening understandings

Mandy Stanley and Shoba Nayar

The purpose of this chapter is to take forward the conversation we started in Chapter 1 and explore several key points in greater depth: (1) differentiating between epistemology, methodology, and methods; (2) researcher positioning and reflexivity; and (3) researcher and research context.

We have chosen the first two key points based on our experience in researching, teaching, reviewing, and editing qualitative studies. Often, students and novice researchers grapple with the new concepts and the nuances of language used in qualitative research, in particular the terms epistemology, methodology, and methods. The confusion of terms is compounded when the choices are not made explicit or the use of language is conflicting within the published literature. A second area of debate, which often flows on from epistemology, is the critique of qualitative research in terms of subjectivity. Thus, we want to discuss the issue of researcher positioning and reflexivity, and the importance of making the researcher's position evident within the research.

Lastly, we turn to the third key point of researcher and research context. In reading through Chapters 3 to 14, it is evident that there are many ways of approaching a qualitative study. In this increasingly changing digital world, researchers may choose to undertake studies on their own, with a team, across countries or to connect more globally through the use of social media. Hence, in rounding out this chapter we pay attention to some of the issues that researchers need to consider when undertaking qualitative research in different contexts, beginning with thinking very close to 'home', then expanding the discussion to researching in 'unfamiliar territory' and utilizing emerging technologies.

However, before addressing the above points, we begin the chapter with an overview of qualitative research in occupational science and occupational therapy, as it has evolved over time. We believe that this is an important place to start to set the context for the forthcoming discussion.

Situating qualitative research in occupational science and occupational therapy

As highlighted in Chapter 1, we sought to develop a text that brought together the richness of qualitative research across both occupational science and occupational therapy. This desire stemmed from our belief in the alignment of qualitative research principles and the aim of occupational science and occupational therapy research being to understand the place of occupation within and throughout people's lives and in the community and society. There is a resonance between the aim of occupational therapy, in working with people to engage in meaningful occupations, and the ability of qualitative research to explore meaning or how people make sense of the world. The discipline of occupational science seeks to better understand the role of engaging in occupations in everyday life, and qualitative approaches provide an array of ways of accessing that kind of information (Carlson & Clark, 1991) – information that cannot be enumerated or captured by measurement without losing some of the richness and depth of meaning. Thus, it is unsurprising that the vast majority of research conducted within occupational science and occupational therapy, to date, is of a qualitative nature.

That said, tracking the history of when occupational therapy researchers started to use qualitative approaches proved more difficult than we imagined! Online searching and indexing tools that are extensively used today do not reach back to the early beginnings of occupational therapy journals. Hence, unless someone performs the laborious task of hand searching (which unfortunately we did not have the resources to do), we are unable to say definitively when the first qualitative studies appeared in the professional literature. It appears that some of the early work came out of the University of Chicago Illinois, in the United States, a university department well known for its strength in scholarship and theory development, as well as qualitative research practices.

From our perspective, Gary Kielhofner and Cheryl Mattingly were among the early pioneers of qualitative research in the occupational therapy profession. In 1982, Kielhofner's review of qualitative methodologies indicated that the use of qualitative research in health care fields was not wide spread. Nearly a decade later, Mattingly (1991) published her seminal work on clinical reasoning making comparisons with the phenomenological tradition. However, both Kielhofner and Mattingly, as with Carlson and Clark (1991), noted that the qualitative research tradition emerged largely from the disciplines of sociology and anthropology. Indeed, much pioneering work in terms of the development of qualitative research methodologies in health was carried out by nurse researchers and has been used to inform occupational therapy research.

Tracking the development of qualitative research within occupational science is somewhat easier. In 1990, Yerxa and colleagues named a variety of research approaches they believed were suited for the study of occupation. Although no rationale was offered for their selection, that list includes commonly used qualitative research methodologies such as ethnography, life history, naturalistic inquiry, and case method. In the early days of using qualitative approaches within occupational therapy, ethnographic studies were the most common. Overtime, that research broadened to include the use of phenomenology – mirroring movements in nursing research. Recently, we have seen the growth of methodologies such as grounded theory and action research. In 1993, the *Journal of Occupational Science* was launched (known as *Journal of Occupational Science: Australia* in the beginning). Many of the earlier publications were theoretical in nature, and early time use studies were quantitative (Pentland, Harvey, & Walker, 1998; Stanley, 1995); however, predominantly the studies published in the *Journal of Occupational Science* are qualitative.

From the beginning of occupational science and occupational therapy, there has been substantial growth in the variety of qualitative methodologies being used, though much of the early work did not differentiate the research design and was simply labeled a qualitative study. However, as Frank and Polkinghorne (2010) discussed, that is no longer acceptable. Hence, we turn to our first key discussion point.

Differentiating between epistemology, methodology and methods

Engaging with any new body of knowledge or undertaking any new skill requires learning a new language particular to that area, and it is no different with qualitative research. While there are a number of terms to become familiar with – many of which will be introduced in the chapters that follow – there are three in particular that apply across the different approaches; these are epistemology, methodology, and methods. At this point, it is important to acknowledge that the terms are often used interchangeably when in fact they mean different things. Alternatively, we have seen authors simply avoid defining or using these terms altogether. Although they are intricately linked, it is important to know the difference between the terms; thus throughout the following chapters, a key aim is to ensure congruence in how they are used. This particular aim emanated from our shared concern of reading published qualitative studies that did not clearly explicate the methodology and appeared to have little understanding of epistemology and how that plays out in the conduct of a study. This speaks back to the call from Frank and Polkinghorne (2010) for a better understanding of the difference between methods and theory and the place of theory in guiding the approach.

Before we define epistemology, methodology, and methods, we refer you to Textbox 2.1 and ask you to pause a moment to consider the reflection questions posed. The purpose of this reflection exercise is to make you start thinking, if you have not done so already, about how you make sense of the terms. Consider writing your responses in a reflective journal as a way of crystallizing your thinking and to be able to revisit your thoughts at a later time in your development as a qualitative researcher or consumer.

Textbox 2.1   Reflection exercise

1   What am I aiming to understand?
2   What kind of knowledge am I seeking to gain?
3   What is my role as the researcher in this study?
4   How do I make sense of the world?

Having spent a few minutes thinking about, and writing your answers to, the questions above, read the definitions below and review your answers.

Epistemology, we consider, is the way of knowing the world and how knowledge is constructed. The epistemological stance taken by the researcher will influence the entire process of the study and the outcome; hence, it is important to be clear about one's epistemology before embarking on a research project. It is not something that can be determined at the end, in retrospect, or even half way through. Eventually, we have come to know ourselves and our shared personal preferences for an understanding of processes. For example, we both like to engage in a consultative process of decision making rather than being given a predetermined outcome. Such a worldview plays out in our everyday work, and in our writing and our thinking, as illustrated by a recent writing project where we combined our grounded theory studies to produce a journal manuscript on occupational adaptation as a social process in everyday life (Nayar & Stanley, 2014). Although these studies were conducted separately for our doctorates, our preferred ways of knowing the world and our views of how knowledge is constructed meant that we could bridge the two studies to highlight a bigger process at play.

Methodology is the theoretical or philosophical orientation. A change in orientation will change the process and outcome of the study. For example, the outcome of a phenomenological study is to obtain a rich description and/or the meaning of the lived experience compared to, for example, a grounded theory study where the outcome is to derive a theory of a social process. Within each of these approaches the theoretical orientation might be drawn from a range of theorists, for example phenomenology may draw on the works of Husserl, Heiddeger, or Gadamer, the grounded theory study from symbolic interactionism or social constructivism. Again, it is important that researchers clearly articulate their theoretical or philosophical orientation as this will help the reader understand how the data were interpreted and the findings were presented, as well as be able to judge the rigor of the study.

Methods, then, are the actual tools for implementing the research. It is the detail of the steps taken by the researcher in conducting the study, for example, the steps of recruitment, participant selection, ethical protocols, data collection approach, phases in analysis, and the strategies to implement rigor. The choice of methods will be influenced by the epistemology and methodology.

It is possible, at times, for epistemologies and methods to overlap around different methodologies. For example, a theoretical orientation in symbolic interactionism could inform both grounded theory and ethnography, and interviews are a common data collection technique used across qualitative methodologies. Interviews are a way of engaging with participants to elicit their stories and perspectives regarding particular phenomenon. However, variations exist within interviews, just as there are variations within qualitative research. Thus, the questions that are asked in an interview, and how they are asked, needs to be congruent with the chosen epistemology and methodology; for example, a semistructured phenomenological interview is not the same as a narrative interview. Thus as, Frank and Polkinghorne (2010) noted, it is critical "that the relationship must be re-established between methods and theories" (p. 56), if the aim is to have occupational science and occupational therapy qualitative research to be taken seriously.

By now, we trust that you, the reader, are coming to appreciate the complexity of qualitative research. As researchers, it is imperative that we take ownership of our chosen approach and what it has to offer, along with the appropriate amount of humility, rigor, and robustness! Equally, it is important for readers of qualitative research to be astute critical consumers to judge the quality of the research and its usefulness for practice. To that end, we have included questions for critiquing studies in each chapter. These questions will be useful to readers of qualitative research and to researchers who can critique the robustness of their own application of the methodology, which leads us to our next conversation piece – researcher positioning and reflexivity.

Positioning and reflexivity

One of the critiques of qualitative research is that it is 'subjective' in nature. We believe that one cannot really do qualitative research without engaging as a person; all researchers come to a study with their experience, shaped by their culture and their own views of reality. Therefore, at the outset, we position ourselves by explicitly stating our assumption that qualitative research is a subjective endeavor and that one way in which subjectivity is managed is through explicating the "lens through which every researcher sees her or his research" (Hasselkus, 1997, p. 81). While there are different ways to position oneself according to different methodologies – as will be discussed in upcoming chapters – here we set the scene for our understanding. It is important to bear in mind that keeping in line with the complexity of qualitative research noted thus far, positioning and reflexivity cannot be considered in isolation; they influence each other and the progression and outcome of the study.

Positioning is the process of making explicit one's personal and epistemological beliefs as a researcher. Given the subjective nature of qualitative research, the analysis of data is always going to be filtered through the researcher's lens. If the researcher positions himself or herself, then readers view the research findings, knowing the researcher's lens, and can make their own judgments about the data presented. Positioning oneself is important throughout the study – not just in the final reporting, but at all stages of the research process, from study design to data collection and analysis – as a way of staying open to data that may not have been anticipated. One way of making positioning explicit is in the reporting, and the researchers stating how they came to do the study and how it relates to them personally. For instance, as an Indian woman and an immigrant, Shoba identified closely with the participants in her study and the stories they were sharing (Nayar, Hocking & Giddings, 2012; see Chapter 4).

However, one of the challenges for novice qualitative researchers is that positioning is not always evident in publications. Journal requirements, such as word limits, may stymie the opportunity to report one's positioning. Yet it is possible to position oneself in a sentence or two, as Shoba did in reporting her study (Nayar et al., 2012). Ensuring the participants and readers of her research knew Shoba was an Indian immigrant women herself was important in both enabling the women to talk openly and assisting the readers to understand what it was the women were sharing in their stories.

Being conscious of and explicitly positioning oneself as a researcher requires an ability to engage in thinking and writing reflexively. Reflexivity can be defined as "the capacity of any system of signification to turn back upon itself, to make itself its own object by referring to itself" (Myerhoff & Ruby, 1992, p. 307). It is the notion that a person's thoughts and ideas tend to be inherently biased; in other words, the values and thoughts of a researcher will be represented in his or her work. Thus, reflexivity is "consciousness about being conscious, thinking about thinking" (Frank, 1997, p. 87). It is a process that goes beyond reflecting on what worked or did not work to questioning and challenging oneself, particularly around assumptions. The aim is to gain a deeper level of insight than previously existed. Using reflexivity will enable a researcher to get new and richer insights. The challenge is not to remove the subjective nature of qualitative research and be free of bias rather to use it as the focus for more intense insight.

Reflexivity may be personal or epistemological in nature. Personal reflexivity encompasses a researcher's values, beliefs, interests, and relationships and how these influence the study. Depending on the topic, there is the potential for reflexivity to take a more psychodynamic lens with a view to transference and counter transference. If it is a topic that is very close to one's personal experience, such as Shoba's description above, then there could be greater risk for issues of transference to occur. At the outset of a study, a researcher may be more focussed on personal reflexivity, whereas epistemological reflexivity may come later in the process. Epistemological reflexivity is the attempt to identify the foundations of knowledge and the implications of any findings. This level of reflexivity adds a further layer of robustness to the study.

We recommend that before engaging in a study, the researcher undertakes a prestudy interview with an experienced qualitative researcher to uncover potential assumptions or understandings related to the field of study. Alternatively, the researcher may wish to journal, reflecting on those questions raised in Textbox 2.2.

Textbox 2.2   Questions to ask for reflexive purposes

1   What do I think I might find in this study?
2   What is my interest in undertaking this study?
3   What current knowledge do I have about this topic?
4   What do I want the outcome of this study to be?
5   Why is it necessary to undertake this study?
6   How am I influencing the gathering and analysis of data?
7   What are the power differentials between me as the researcher and those I am researching?
8   Am I being true to the epistemology and methodology of the study?

Whatever strategy one chooses to use, it is important to remember that reflexivity is not just thinking about assumptions, it is an active process of writing, talking, asking, and questioning until the researcher encounters the 'aha' moment through examining the origins of his or her assumptions.

A further issue to consider is that of ethics and power in the partnership between researcher and participant or participant groups. We believe it is not ethical to approach a qualitative study with the 'drive by' or 'hit and run' idea of engaging briefly with participants, doing the research, and then exiting to write up the thesis or publication with no intention of making contact again. Taking that approach reduces the likelihood of accessing participants who are willing to share their experiences. On the other hand, some people may volunteer to participate in the study, but given the lack of acknowledgement of the contribution and reciprocity, the next researcher who comes along is not going to be received well. As researchers, it is important for the discipline and the profession to make a positive contribution in participants' lives and an equally useful contribution to knowledge; however, this requires that researchers are aware of sensitivities in negotiations with prospective participants and dissemination of findings. Thus, in the spirit of doing justice to both participants and methodological rigor, it is important to consider the research context and potential issues of power that may influence the study. Suggestions for reflexive questions to stimulate thinking about relationships with participants are shown in Figure 2.1.

An astute reader will identify that we have stated our position in Chapter 1 as editors and how we came to this text. Each of the authors have explicated their positioning in relation to the methodology – which you will see is a common feature of all chapters in this book. The purpose is to provide the reader with

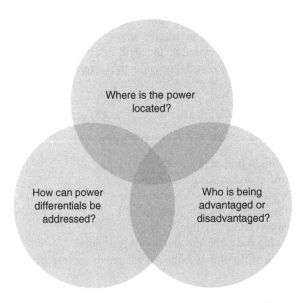

Figure 2.1 Reflexive questions in relation to power differentials

examples of how to frame one's positioning, as well as ensuring that we are being rigorous and true to what we are recommending as good practice.

Research context

Having considered issues of language, positioning, and reflexivity, this section explores some of the varied contexts within which qualitative studies can be conducted, and the strengths, challenges, and implications. To frame this section we draw on the image of concentric circles with the researcher placed in the very center. The discussion begins with research in close personal contexts before moving to more unfamiliar contexts, including engaging in multisite studies in multiple countries and extending out to address the emergence of digital technologies (see Figure 2.2).

Close personal context

More often than not, people come to research with a question (or multiple questions) either from practice or from their lived experience. If it is a question from

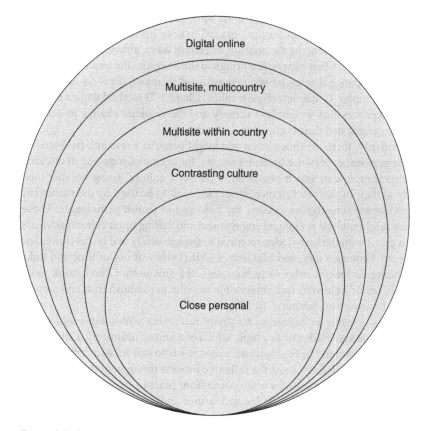

Figure 2.2 Contexts for conducting qualitative research

practice, the researcher already has a body of knowledge from his or her education, reading, and practice experiences with clients or colleagues. Thus, as indicated above, it is impossible to enter the research field free of assumptions. Equally, if a person comes to a question from personal experience, the drive to pursue that question is because it has personal meaning, which again is accompanied by a set of assumptions based on that experience; thus, it is more of an embodied experience and comes with a different set of knowledge.

A balance is required in terms of having the drive and personal interest to pursue a question and, at the same time, recognizing the underlying assumptions and values, and how they might impact the choice of methodology and methods used in the research. It is harder to reveal one's own assumptions and values if researching something closely related to personal experience. It is much harder to separate out the cognitive and emotive elements, and the researcher will be naturally drawn to focus attention on data that speak of his or her own experience. For instance, if the researcher's lived experience is of being a refugee who has resettled in a new country and is now involved in research with other refugees about their settlement experiences, it is particularly important to be vigilant in the analysis phase. Data that present alternative experiences to that experienced by the researcher need to be brought forward and the researcher must work hard to incorporate any 'outlier' data. It is much more difficult for the 'insider' to keep his or her own values and assumptions from influencing the analysis in certain ways, although there is much that a researcher with that experience brings to the analysis. For example, Wilson (2010), an occupational scientist and occupational therapist, drew on descriptive qualitative (Chapter 3) and autoethnographic (Chapter 7) methodologies to write about her experience of weight loss surgery and the resultant change in occupational engagement and thus occupational identity.

Alternatively, there are times when one might come to a research field having very little personal experience of the topic area; for example, engaging in research with cultural groups in which one is not a part of ('culture' being broader than ethnicity alone). In such an instance, strategies need to be used by the researcher that demonstrate sensitivities to enter the field and to recruit participants. These strategies might include prolonged engagement and calling upon cultural advisors who can assist with the knowledge required to engage safely and respectfully. For example, in Thomas, Gray, and McGinty's (2012) study of use of time and links to well-being for people who were homeless, the first author "undertook more than 100 hours of fieldwork and observation in order to establish trust and rapport within the homeless community" (p. 784).

Thus, it is possible to engage as a solitary researcher with a topic which one might have little knowledge of to a topic which one knows intimately. Either way, we strongly recommend having another researcher who can act as a critical friend and, using peer debriefing, assist the reflexive process throughout the study.

Given that research questions often come from practice or experience, it may well be that the research study is located within one's own workplace or community, which will impact on who will volunteer and what participants will be prepared to reveal. The researcher has to pay attention to preserving participants' rights to retain confidentiality and be sensitive to the potential for coercion and a sense of obligation to volunteer. Some ways to alleviate the issues might be, in addition to undertaking research as the sole investigator, to engage in research as part of a team or using online methods.

Multisite (within a country and international)

Increasingly, multisite studies are the way forward for many researchers, as funders look towards studies that incorporate multiple perspectives. Multisite studies are still relatively uncommon within the fields of occupational science and occupational therapy; however, we are starting to see, as part of the maturation of the discipline and profession, the bringing together of research teams that add further layers of complexity to the research process. Multisite studies entail both richness and challenges; for example, having multiple perspectives or 'lenses' through which to view the data may result in deeper insights, with relevance of research findings beyond that of one profession.

Alternatively, researcher positioning and reflexivity may pose a challenge if researchers' personal and epistemological perspectives to do not align among members of the team. Therefore, key to engaging in a multisite study is the researcher's ability to be a good communicator and willingness and commitment to engage in robust frank conversations, in a collaborative process, in order for the desired outcomes to be achieved, cultural values respected, and relationships preserved. Working effectively in teams is facilitated by clear documentation of team decisions, particularly in relation to ownership of data and what it can be used for, as well as agreements about allocation of tasks, timelines, intellectual property, publication and authorship.

Multisite studies within a country might be undertaken as a very strategic approach to increasing the chances of recruiting participants from different regions, as well as achieving sufficient participant numbers. Additionally, the findings from multisite studies in the same country will hold broader application of outcome and transferability. The researchers will make a commitment to answering the same research questions and following the grant proposal or agreed protocols. The added complexity for researchers then is quite pragmatic about methods of communication across geographical locations, and possibly accounting for some time zone differences in countries like Canada, Australia, and the United States. When it comes to multicountry research, complexities are amplified. Working across more distant geographies brings additional challenges through different language and culture, time zones, institutional requirements for governance and ethics, governments, legislative requirements, and politics. With both of these configurations of multisite research, additional time needs to be spent prior to writing the research proposal to engage in shared discussions about ways of working and epistemological positioning (Shoredike et al., 2010).

Within occupational science there are few examples of multisite studies, the most well-known being the food-centered occupations study conducted in New Zealand, Thailand, and the United States. Findings from the site-specific studies have been published separately (Shoredike & Pierce, 2005; Wright-St Clair, Bunrayong, Vittayakorn, Rattakorn, & Hocking, 2004) and in combination (Wright-St Clair et al., 2013), along with a methodology paper (Shoredike et al., 2010). Further discussion of the methodologies and processes that promote successful crosscultural research in occupational science and occupational therapy is urgently required.

Researchers should also be aware of emerging discussions around decolonizing methodologies for studying topics involving indigenous groups (Tuhiwai Smith, 2012). Similar to the lead taken by feminist researchers in the 1970s, the use of decolonizing methodologies places the disadvantaged group into a 'privileged' position epistemologically and ethically to protect the groups' interests and prevent further oppression or marginalization. Amidst calls for occupational science research to broaden its exploration away from a Western focus, these methodologies warrant further investigation.

Emergence of online research

We turn now to thinking about research in contexts that defy geographical boundaries. The growth in the use of online and social media provides exciting opportunities for researching, both in terms of people engaging in occupations online, as well as the place of online or social media in the lives of clients of occupational therapy practice and the use of online tools for conducting research and for generating research data. Use of digital media facilitates multisite research activities by providing tools to assist the way researchers work enabling better communication. In this short section, we do not propose to provide extensive coverage of all the different types of tools or applications nor do we have anything to gain from mentioning some products and not others, rather our intention is to talk more broadly about the ways that media might be used. Researchers now have access to free or inexpensive applications as long as there is a computer, tablet or mobile device with good Internet connection. Tools such as Skype® can be used to talk to colleagues in real time in different geographical locations, and if participants have a webcam it is possible to see each other as well, which is important for the nonverbal aspects of communication. Other tools furnished by the Internet for storage and exchange of files (e.g., Dropbox, iCloud) and sharing bibliographic databases (Refworks, Endnote web) all provide ways to make the work of multisite research easier. The tools just mentioned are available 24 hours a day, which is useful when working across diverse time zones.

The use of online forums, blogs, and social media provides researchers with a ready source of data, much of which is freely available in the public domain. While the emergence of online research presents increasing options for accessing data, such exciting opportunities raise a need for caution, including the need to pause and consider the ethics associated with undertaking research where participants may not be willingly or knowingly consenting to having their ideas used for research when they write a blog or send a tweet. Ethical issues arise around informed consent, or the lack of it, the inability to gain informed consent from the writer of the information and the inability to return to the originator of the material and check the researcher's interpretations.

It appears that there is scant literature in occupational science or occupational therapy on Internet-based qualitative research. Within qualitative health research, Wilkerson, Iantaffi, Grey, Bockting, and Rosser (2014) have provided researchers with two checklists: one for deciding between the use of online or offline data collection and the second to guide decision making about when to begin online data collection. Drawing on their experience, with several qualitative projects with hard-to-read groups on sensitive topics, they offer a useful discussion on the use of online forums for recruiting and data collection. However, there is little guidance available on the use of other social media, hence the need for methodological literature from the perspective of occupational science or occupational therapy research.

Summary

In this chapter, our conversation has taken us back in time to briefly overview the history of qualitative research in occupational science and occupational therapy; and we have chosen three key issues to explore that underpin all qualitative research: differentiating between epistemology, methodology, and methods; researcher positioning and reflexivity; and research context. While we raise these as topics for conversation, it is not all that can be talked about. However, it is also not our intention to expand and replicate in this textbook what can be found elsewhere. We suggest that people seek out the abundant literature that is now readily accessible online and refer to further readings and websites at the end of this and subsequent chapters in the book.

Qualitative research is not always what it appears to be; thus it is important to emphasize the need to see beyond what one is told. Qualitative research is not formulaic. It is highly complex, evolving, and exciting. The following chapters further the conversation we have started here to reveal the creativity, complexity and richness that is qualitative research.

References

Carlson, M. E., & Clark, F. A. (1991). The search for useful methodologies in occupational science. *American Journal of Occupational Therapy, 45*(3), 235–241.

Frank, G. (1997). Is there life after categories? Reflexivity in qualitative research. *Occupational Therapy Journal of Research, 17*(2), 84–98.

Frank, G., & Polkinghorne, D. (2010). Qualitative research in occupational therapy: From the first to the second generation. *OTJR Occupation, Participation and Health, 30*(2), 51–57. doi:10.3928/15394492–20100325–02.

Hasselkus, B. R. (1997). In the eye of the beholder: The researcher in qualitative research. *Occupational Therapy Journal of Research, 17*(2), 81–83.

Kielhofner, G. (1982). Qualitative research: Part one paradigmatic grounds and issues of reliability and validity. *American Journal of Occupational Therapy, 2*(2), 67–79.

Mattingly, C. (1991). What is clinical reasoning? *American Journal of Occupational Therapy, 45*(11), 979–986.

Myerhoff, B., & Ruby, J. (1982/1992). A crack in the mirror: Reflexive perspectives in anthropology. In B. Myerhoff (Ed.), *Remembered lives: The work of ritual, storytelling, and growing older* (pp. 307–340). Ann Arbor, MI: University of Michigan Press.

Nayar, S., Hocking, C., & Giddings, L. (2012). Using occupation to navigate cultural spaces: Indian immigrant women settling in New Zealand. *Journal of Occupational Science, 19*(1), 62–75. doi:10.1080/14427591.2011.602628.

Nayar, S., & Stanley, M. (2014). Occupational adaptation as a social process in everyday life. *Journal of Occupational Science.* doi:10.1080/14427591.2014.882251.

Pentland, W., Harvey, A., & Walker, J. (1998). The relationship between time use and health and well-being in men with spinal cord injury. *Journal of Occupational Science, 5*(1), 14–25.

Shoredike A., Hocking, C., Pierce, D., Wright-St Clair, V., Vittayakorn, S., Rattakorn, P., & Bunrayong, W. (2010). Respecting regional culture in an international multi-site study: A derived etic method. *Qualitative Research, 10*(3), 333–355. doi:10.1177/1468794109369145.

Shoredike, A., & Pierce, D. (2005). Cooking up Christmas in Kentucky: Occupation and tradition in the stream of time. *Journal of Occupational Science, 12*, 140–148.

Stanley, M. (1995). An investigation into the relationship between engagement in valued occupations and life satisfaction for elderly South Australians. *Journal of Occupational Science: Australia, 2*(3), 100–114.

Thomas, Y., Gray, M., & McGinty, S. (2012). An exploration of subjective wellbeing among people experiencing homelessness: A strengths-based approach. *Social Work in Health Care, 51*, 780–797. doi:10.1080/00981389.2012.686475.

Tuhiwai Smith, L. (2012). *Decolonizing methodologies: Research and indigenous peoples* (2nd ed.). London, UK: Zed Books.

Wilkerson, J. M., Iantaffi, A., Grey, J., Bockting, W., & Rosser, B. R. S. (2014). Recommendations for internet-based qualitative health research with hard-to-reach populations. *Qualitative Health Research, 24*(4), 561–574. doi:10.1177/1049732314524635.

Wilson, L. (2010). Occupational consequences of weight loss surgery: A personal reflection. *Journal of Occupational Science, 17*(1), 47–54. doi:10.1080/14427591.2010.9686672.

Wright-St Clair, V., Bunrayong, W., Vittayakorn, S., Rattakorn, P., & Hocking, C. (2004). Offerings: Food traditions of older Thai women at Songkran. *Journal of Occupational Science, 11*, 115–124.

Wright-St Clair, V., Pierce, D., Bunrayong, W., Rattakorn, P, Vittayakorn, S., Shoredike, A., & Hocking, C. (2013). Cross-cultural understandings of festival food-related activities for older women in Chiang Mai, Thailand, Eastern Kentucky, USA, and Auckland, New Zealand. *Journal of Cross Cultural Gerontology, 28*(2), 103–119. doi:10.1007/s10823–013–9194–5.

Yerxa, E. J., Clark, F., Frank, G., Jackson, J., Parham, D., Pierce, D., Stein, C., & Zemke, R. (1990). An introduction to occupational science: A foundation for occupational therapy in the 21st century. *Occupational Therapy in Health Care, 6*, 1–17.

Further reading

Denzin, N., & Lincoln, Y. (Eds.). (2005). *The Sage handbook of qualitative research* (3rd ed.). Thousand Oaks, CA: Sage.

Finlay, L., & Gough, B. (2003). *Reflexivity: A practical guide for researchers in health and social sciences.* Oxford, UK: Blackwell Science.

Patton, M. Q. (2002). *Qualitative research and evaluation methods* (3rd ed.). Thousand Oaks, CA: Sage.

Website

http://www.nova.edu/ssss/QR/qualres.html

3 Qualitative descriptive

A very good place to start

Mandy Stanley

With this first methodological chapter, I begin with the most exploratory generic approach to qualitative research: qualitative descriptive. It is the least sophisticated approach with regards to epistemological stance as there is no alignment to a particular theoretical orientation. However, just because it is generic and the least theoretically sophisticated, do not mistakenly think it is simple! When novices begin their foray into the world of qualitative research, this is often the approach chosen as there is possibly a less steep learning curve than some of the methodological approaches that follow in later chapters. However, the elegant simplicity of a quality study belies the thinking and planning required for data collection, analysis, and presentation of the findings.

Notwithstanding, a descriptive qualitative approach is a good place for novices to "cut their teeth" with a generic approach to the design and conduct of a qualitative study. Equally, more experienced researchers find that the approach meets their needs for a pragmatic design that yields rich data and has the ability to reveal taken for granted ideas. Many of the techniques are used in other methodological approaches (as seen in later chapters), but with greater attention paid to the theoretical underpinnings of the methodology. In this chapter, I draw on my experience of conducting a number of studies using a descriptive qualitative methodology, including a funded study with a team of researchers in which we explored older people's and service providers' understandings of loneliness (Stanley et al., 2010).

I use this particular methodological approach frequently in my work with occupational therapy honors students and share their frustration in struggling to find literature that guides them in how to go about planning and conducting a rigorous qualitative descriptive study. In my work as an occupational therapy academic reviewing manuscripts for journals and in my role as an associate editor of the *Journal of Occupational Science*, I am often dismayed by studies that purport to be qualitative descriptive yet lack rigor in their application of the approach. Therefore, in this chapter I seek to contribute to the literature on descriptive qualitative methodology and provide guidance to researchers utilizing the approach.

Background

The methodology is most often attributed to Sandelowski (2000) after the publication of her article 'Whatever happened to qualitative description?'; however, the term is used to refer to a range of approaches varying in the amount of interpretation. In 2010, Sandelowski wrote to clarify that it was not *her* methodology, rather the intent of the 2000 article was to outline the approach. She claimed to have been misinterpreted as she was not arguing that it is purely descriptive without any interpretation: in the act of describing the researcher is already adding interpretation. Approaches to qualitative descriptive could be placed along a continuum of interpretation from low to high. My work and the study referred to in this chapter is probably toward the more interpretive end of the continuum. Wherever a study is placed along that continuum, the outcome will still be a rich description and not theory.

Sandelowski's intention in writing the 2000 article was to address the issue of researchers stating that they were using grounded theory or narrative or phenomenology and clearly were not. While this critique was leveled at nursing research, it could equally have applied to occupational therapy. Some of the earliest occupational therapy qualitative studies published claim to draw on phenomenology (Kibele & Llorens, 1989) or do not state the research design (Merrill, 1985); however, they appear to be qualitative descriptive studies.

Epistemology

While there is no specific philosophy or theory guiding the approach, it is not atheoretical, and the occupational science or occupational therapy researcher can look to authors such as Sandelowski (2000) and Thorne, Kirkham, and O'Flynn-Magee (2004) who convincingly argued for the place of qualitative descriptive studies in health research rather than it being considered as 'the poor cousin' (Neergaard, Olesen, Andersen, & Sondergaard, 2009).

Aside from any debates about the amount of interpretation, a qualitative descriptive methodology fits within an interpretive paradigm (Denzin & Lincoln, 2005). The methodology provides a way of studying people in their context and how they make sense of the world with a subjectivist epistemology and a relativist ontology (Guba & Lincoln, 2005). The very pragmatic approach is a good fit for many occupational scientists and occupational therapists.

Positioning

Given the epistemology, it is important to clearly position myself as a researcher and how I came to the study. Just after I completed my PhD, I was invited to join a team submitting a grant application about loneliness to a national funding body. I came to the project with a strong clinical background in all aspects of aged care, a passion for researching what enables older people to live well and some experience in small-scale qualitative studies.

The loneliness study was situated in aged care service provision rather than in occupational science or occupational therapy; however, I believed that I would be able to view the findings within an occupational framework which was far easier than I imagined due to the very occupational nature of the data itself. The team of researchers working on the grant was multidisciplinary made up of a sociologist, nurse researchers, aged care administrators and my contribution as an occupational science/occupational therapy researcher. I relished the opportunity to be part of a team with other experienced qualitative researchers and industry partners working on a large project.

Defining the topic and formulating the question

There is much debate about the place of the literature in a qualitative study and the extent to which a literature review is conducted prior to doing the study. Some authors argue that doing an extensive literature review has too much influence on the data collection and the analysis, so there is a danger that the researcher will find what is already known and not be open to the unknown or unexpected (Creswell, 2007). However, granting bodies and research ethics committees will not approve studies that do not have a review of literature which clearly establishes the gap in knowledge that the proposed study aims to address and a strong rationale for why a qualitative approach is the right choice for the study. Therefore, the literature review is important. The researcher needs to be able to situate his or her study within the literature and be sensitized to what is already known but be open to new, unforeseen or unexpected data.

The decision to study loneliness and older people arose from a workshop conducted with an industry partner to generate potential research topics that were needed in the field and matched the interests and expertise of the researchers. Gaining 'real' collaboration with the industry partner and "buy in" not only with money to conduct the study but with genuine interest and cooperation is facilitated by working on a 'real' problem in the everyday world of the industry partner. When we turned to the literature about loneliness, we found that as a concept it was not well understood; loneliness was conflated with social isolation, there was mounting evidence that loneliness is associated with significant ill health effects, little evidence of successful interventions, and importantly, the perspective of the older person, and of service providers themselves, was largely absent. These key points provided a very strong argument for the study, and for using a descriptive qualitative approach. Therefore, the 'Alone in a Crowd' study sought to answer the research question "What are older people's and service providers' perspectives on loneliness for older people?" Other examples of research questions from published occupational science and occupational therapy studies are included in Table 3.1.

According to Patton (2002), a qualitative descriptive approach is well suited to program evaluation research. Corresponding research questions might be: "What do the clients think of this service?" "What are service users' perspectives?" The aim is to seek the view or perspective of a sample group, such as occupational therapists' descriptions of their work with persons who had acquired brain injury and were experiencing cognitive impairment (Holmqvist et al., 2009) or occupational therapists' perceptions of their participation in different modalities for maintenance of professional currency (Murray & Lawry, 2011).

Table 3.1 Examples of research questions studied with a qualitative descriptive methodology

---

How do Swedish occupational therapists describe their work with persons with cognitive impairment from acquired brain injury? (Holmqvist, Kamwendo, & Ivasrsson, 2009)

What are the perspectives of students and clinical educators of 1:1 and 2:1 models of clinical education across occupational therapy and physiotherapy programs? (O'Connor, Cahill, & McKay, 2012)

What is the nature of routines in the family when a person is affected by mental illness? (Koome, Hocking, & Sutton, 2012)

Sampling and recruitment

The researcher can draw on different types of purposive sampling, depending on the topic and question, as well as pragmatics of whom one can access, time, finances, and location. Furthermore, it is important to remember that this type of research does not require a representative sample. Given the broad scope for sampling in this approach, it is important that the researcher provide specific details of the type of sampling used. Patton (2002) outlined 15 different types of purposive sampling and the logic behind them which provide guidance to the researcher about the type of purposive sampling to suit the purpose of their study. Making a considered choice about sampling will enhance the rigor of the study.

In the loneliness study, we used maximum variation sampling. The logic behind the decision was that 'older people' are a very large population and they are not a homogenous group, and we were looking to explore the variation around the phenomenon of loneliness. Therefore, we wanted to recruit men and women as loneliness could be a gendered experience – from a range of living situations (community, residential, alone, with a partner or with others), a range of geographical locations, a range of ages and health status, and backgrounds. We were not after equal numbers for each characteristic of variation; thus we established a sampling frame to guide recruitment and ensure that our sample showed the variation in the experience of the phenomenon (refer to Table 3.2 for various aspects of the sampling frame). The older people did not have to be lonely but needed to be able to talk about their perceptions of what loneliness was for older people.

It is important also to think about the sites for data collection and sampling in relation to those sites. Guided by purposive sampling, South Australia and Queensland

Table 3.2 Sampling frame for 'Alone in a Crowd' study

Age	Gender	Living status	Marital status
65 years through to 90+	Male	Alone/with partner/with family	Married
	Female	Own home/rental	Widowed
		Residential aged care facility high/low care	Single (divorced, never married)

were chosen as information-rich sites for the study because of their rapid growth in the proportion of people aged 65 and above (Australian Bureau of Statistics, 2009). The industry partners in each state are large providers of care and services to older people, including retirement living, long-term and community care in their respective states, and were selected using the strategy of typical site purposive sampling, in that they were "not in any major way atypical, extreme, deviant, or intensely unusual" (Patton, 2002, p. 236). These organizations compare in size, structure, and remit to most other major providers of aged care services in Australia.

Participants were recruited through advertising in newsletters and flyers, as well as through key contacts within each of the industry partner organizations. In total, 60 older people participated in in-depth interviews. Key contacts also recruited support and service providers for the focus groups from within their aged care organizations and the local community. Focus groups were held in both metropolitan and rural areas, with the rural areas chosen for being regional centers and having high numbers of older people. Lists of possible participants were drawn together, ensuring that a diverse range of service providers and support workers were invited to participate.

Participants included nurses and personal care assistants working in the collaborating aged care organizations, other health professionals who were associated with the study site in the provision of support and services, managers of those providing direct care and/or support services, directors responsible for allocating resources in aged care industry, family members/significant others of older people receiving support/services from aged care industry, and representatives of consumer groups. Four focus groups were held in each State in metropolitan and rural areas with approximately 10 people attending each group. Determining sample size is influenced by the pragmatics of the funding available and the size of the population the sample can be drawn from. Researchers' decisions about the appropriate sample size can be guided by exemplars in the literature of published studies that have undergone peer review drawing on similar populations.

Data collection

The primary sources of data in a qualitative descriptive study are likely to be semistructured in-depth interviews; however, it is also possible to use the methods of observation and document analysis in this approach. Interview questions are broad and open-ended to elicit a rich response, but it is surprising how easy it is to slip back into asking closed questions. Many readers will be familiar with asking focused questions in their work with people to access accurate information in as short a time as possible; however, research interviewing is quite different. One line of questioning I have found helpful is to encourage participants to think about someone outside of themselves, for instance an interview question might be "If you were talking to your daughter on the phone, how would you describe the service?" It is a good idea to have a concluding question "Is there anything I have not asked about with regard to X that you would like to tell me about?" to elicit material that was not anticipated.

The researcher also needs to have a store of probing questions at the ready to extend responses and to assist participants to articulate their experience. Examples of probing questions are provided in Textbox 3.1.

Textbox 3.1   Examples of the types and format of probing questions (Gillham, 2000)

Clarifying:	I don't quite understand that, can you explain it to me?
Showing understanding:	How did you feel about that?
Justifying:	What makes you say that?
Relevance:	You've lost me, how do those two things connect?
Asking for an example:	What do you mean by . . . ? Can you give me an example?
Extending the narrative:	Tell me more about that.
Accuracy:	Now, let me see if I've got things in the right order?

Two different approaches to data collection were taken in the Alone in a Crowd study. First, we used semistructured in-depth interviews to access the older people's perceptions of loneliness. Interviews were conducted by members of the research team in the older person's home or place of residence so that the person felt comfortable in familiar surroundings. To keep the focus of the interview on the topic, an interview guide was developed (Textbox 3.2) and piloted, and less experienced interviewers observed an interview conducted by a more experienced interviewer before conducting interviews on their own. The emphasis here is on the quality of the data that is yielded from the interview rather than consistency, as in essence the interview is a co-construction between the older person and the interviewer. Mishler (1986) contended that the research interview is a joint construction of meaning between the interviewer and the respondent. The richness of qualitative data, and I argue the key contribution, lies in that co-construction.

The setting of an appointment to be interviewed about their views on loneliness will bring an older person to thinking about loneliness which they may not have done without being involved in the research study. The way the questions are phrased and then re-formulated to elicit conversation with the participants and the responses that are forthcoming are shaped by the discourses between the interviewer and the participant. The older people who we interviewed often asked us if what they were saying was what we were after, implying that we had an idea of a correct response. Their responses would have been shaped by the rapport we built and by our reactions to what they were saying.

Interview questions for the in-depth interviews are included in Textbox 3.2. The questions for the interview guide drew on the literature, and the guide was constructed from our experience as qualitative researchers to answer our research question. We conducted 30 interviews in each State resulting in 60 in-depth interviews overall lasting from 17 to 90 minutes. We kept a data sheet for each of the interviews on which the interviewer recorded demographic information such as age, living situation and self-reported health status, as well as the interviewer writing a brief reflection about the interview. The reflection may have included contextual notes and impressions. The choice of using data sheets was to assist us in keeping track of a large number of participants when there were multiple interviews. The strategy may still be useful with one interviewer and a small number of participants but is not a requirement.

Textbox 3.2   Interview and focus group question guide

Tell me about:

- Your perceptions and understandings of loneliness
- What you think contributes to loneliness
- How you think older people manage loneliness
- How you think loneliness impacts on the health and well-being of the older person
- What assists, or could assist, an older person to manage loneliness
- What you think the barriers are to managing loneliness

The second approach to data collection was the use of focus groups to gain the support and service providers' perspectives. This approach to data collection was a good fit for the topic and the sample. We had to be conscious of staff fitting the focus group into their work time and so offered refreshments, and this gave us fairly homogenous groups that could contribute and add to other group members' contributions. Dissenting views were encouraged by the facilitators.

The same interview guide from the in-depth interviews was used for the focus groups. The focus group data was really rich as the participants drew on their experience working with older people as well as their personal experience of older parents and relatives and their own experience of loneliness. We did not record demographic data for participants and in hindsight we should have recorded age, role and length of experience working in aged care in order to describe the sample. Each focus group was run by two members of the team with one facilitating and the other observing, and the reflections were documented.

All interviews and focus groups were digitally recorded and transcribed verbatim by professional transcriptionists. There are pros and cons to using a professional to transcribe rather than transcribing data oneself. If researchers do their own transcription the familiarity with the data is greatly increased; however, it can be very time consuming depending on the speed of typing and access to transcribing equipment or technology. For every 1 hour of recorded interview it can be expected to take 3–4 hours to transcribe or longer depending on the quality of the recording. The time spent has to be balanced with the costs of having transcription done professionally as it can be expensive. Davidson (2009) argued that transcription is theoretical and part of the analysis process and identified a number of issues with utilizing professional transcribers including omission or alteration of words but also offered suggestions for working with professionals.

Data analysis

Analysis is not a linear process as might be indicated by the presentation of steps of analysis in reports or publications. Rather, it is iterative and recursive, as will be evident in most of the chapters in this text. Analysis in qualitative descriptive studies draws on generic approaches, and methods for analysis are not as well articulated as analysis approaches for other methodologies. That said, researchers still need to be able to clearly articulate their analytic pathway, including keeping an audit trail of decisions made. Two approaches to analysis include content analysis and the more indicative interpretive approach of thematic analysis. Both these approaches involve some process of open coding, grouping like codes and then collapsing those grouped codes into themes. Some studies will use the literature to generate a list of start codes for analysis but still remain open to the possibility of the data not fitting these codes and being able to generate new ones. For example, Kosma, Bryant, and Wilson (2013) examined 37 publications and conducted a content analysis using a framework they had constructed from textual analysis of Wilcock's seminal work to ascertain the impact that Wilcock's theoretical work has had within occupational therapy research and practice.

Content analysis

Content analysis involves examining the data for patterns and trends. Liamputtong (2013) suggested that codes for content analysis are predetermined, which means that the researchers already anticipate what they will find in the data. Content analysis is a pragmatic approach to analyzing text which requires little induction and interpretation. It is more akin to counting or looking at the frequency of certain words and phrases occurring in the data. In my opinion, content analysis is a useful analytical approach for short sections of text, for example, responses to open-ended questions on a questionnaire. My preference for analyzing larger amounts of data including data from interviews is thematic analysis. I believe that it is a loss of opportunity to collect rich data to then lose the richness in analysis by using content analysis. Having said that, there is not a shared understanding of what content analysis is and some authors will use the term content analysis to describe what I would term thematic analysis.

Thematic analysis

The thematic analysis needs to be inductive moving through a process of coding in layers of abstraction and interpretation. For example, if the outcome of analysis of a study of maintaining physical exercise following a stroke results in a theme called barriers and another theme facilitators, it is evident that there is very little interpretation and abstraction during analysis. The researcher has to keep working on the analysis to 'lift' it to a more conceptual level without losing the richness of the data to what Thorne and Derbyshire (2005) called "bloodless" findings. One strategy to keep the richness is to draw on participants' words for theme names as Murray and Lawry (2011) have demonstrated with one of the themes about maintaining professional currency being named "You have to have people around you". This theme describes participants' need to feel connected and secure and to validate what they were doing against others as well as the social construction of knowledge through the exchange of ideas.

From my experience of undertaking research and supervising students using this approach, the researcher should aim for a maximum of three to five themes. Too many themes and analysis becomes too thin; fewer themes might indicate not enough data has been gathered. Data analysis should yield a rich description of participants' views on the topic being explored, allowing the reader a better understanding of another's perspective.

The first phase of analysis of the Alone in a Crowd data was conducted by research assistants working on the interview data from each state separately, communicating by telephone and email. They began by reading the interview through in its entirety, then open coding line by line. At this stage, the analysis stays fairly close to the participants' words and may well use 'in vivo' codes, that is, the language of the participants (see Textbox 3.3).

Textbox 3.3   Example of open coding of the transcript

Verbatim text	*Open coding*
It is difficult to explain. If I am sewing then I am concentrating on something else and I am fine. Doing the vacuuming, washing up or anything like that, then you don't have time to think about the lack of conversation, lack of discussing events, lack of arguing.	*Hard to explain and talk about* *Doing activities helps to distract from thinking about things that are missing in life*

Following open coding, similar codes were brought together to form categories. Analysis continued with the researchers discussing each category, debating the place of data and suggesting moves. We used a manual process which included writing the codes onto sticky notes and attaching them to large sheets of paper on the wall so that the data could clearly be seen and easily moved around as we progressed through our iterative process.

It was at this stage that the data from the two states were brought together. There were some small differences in the two data sets with the South Australian data including a few more multicultural participants and the Queensland data being stronger in stoicism for the rural participants; however, we considered these differences were not enough to stop us from combining the data sets. A similar process of analysis of the individual interviews was conducted with the focus group data. Further data analysis resulted in a collection of what at this stage we called themes. It was then that we had an 'aha' moment. The most experienced qualitative researcher of the group suggested that what we had was not separate themes but rather dimensions of loneliness. We were dimensionalizing the concept of loneliness compared to describing recurring ideas as themes. This was a key point in our data analysis and helped us shift from a more descriptive level to a conceptual level. The usual outcome of a thematic analysis is to generate themes, so there were some grounded theory influences to our analysis reflecting Sandelowski's (2000) notion of hues, tones and textures from other approaches. See Table 3.3 where I list early themes from our analysis and link them to the five dimensions that we derived at the end of analysis.

The five dimensions of loneliness were private, relational, (dis)connectedness, temporal, and adjustment. The adjustment dimension came from the focus group data only and we puzzled about this. This dimension is about the adjustment to the challenges in life that come with aging. It seemed to make sense that the dimension about adjustment might be identified by workers who were external to the process and saw large numbers of older people in their work, rather than by individuals.

Having team members from different disciplines added to the strength of our study but posed challenges to work through in analysis. Each of us came to data analysis with a particular 'lens' which was colored by our experience in aged care and our immersion in the language and knowledge of own discipline. Robust discussion occurred during data analysis to work through the differences and arrive at consensus. For example, we debated use of the word 'depression' to label a theme. For some members of the team the label of 'depression' was too closely aligned to a biomedical model being imposed on the data and could be taken to imply a diagnosis drawing on accepted clinical criteria which we were unable to validate with the participants themselves. We preferred to use terms such as 'feelings associated with grief and loss' that conveyed the content but did not have quite the same clinical associations. In another example, when the academics doing the analysis presented the temporal dimension to our industry partners, there was some confusion. Temporal in this sense was used in relation to time, where older people moved in and out of loneliness at different times of the day, week, season, lifespan; loneliness was not necessarily a defining feature of an older person's life. However, our industry partners thought we were referring to the temporal lobe of the brain and were having difficulty working out the link with the data on loneliness. Even when we were using the same words we needed to

Table 3.3 Contrasting descriptive themes from early analysis with conceptual dimensions

Theme	Dimension
Hard to describe	Private
Stigma associated	
Family is important	Relational
Connections: maintaining old, making new	(dis)Connectedness
Shaped by context	Temporal
Adjusting to loss	Readjustment

work to make sure each member of the team had a shared understanding of what we were discussing.

Rigor/ethics

Given the broad nature of the qualitative descriptive approach, the researcher may use a range of strategies to establish rigor and trustworthiness. These strategies include journaling to provide a clear audit trail of methodological decisions made during the research process, member checking, peer debriefing including supervision or discussion with a more experienced qualitative researcher, as well as presentations to a range of audiences including colleagues and research stakeholders. With a large variety of strategies available, it is advisable for the researcher to be selective and choose strategies that best demonstrate the rigor of the study in depth.

Some of the strategies to ensure rigor in the Alone in a Crowd study have already been described as I have laid out the data collection and analysis process we undertook, for example, the peer debriefing. Another key strategy for rigor was the use of triangulation. We triangulated data with the use of both interviews and focus groups, and triangulation of researchers with multiple data collectors. We kept an audit trail of the project through team meeting minutes, in addition to keeping different versions of the analysis as it progressed to document the methodological and analytical decision made along the way.

Member checking is a common rigor strategy for descriptive qualitative studies where the researcher returns to the participants at various points to check the accuracy of interpretations of the data. One often reads of researchers taking transcripts back to participants for checking the accuracy of the transcription. In my opinion there are more useful times to use member checking if you have digitally recorded the interview, transcribed verbatim, and checked the accuracy of the transcription against the digital recording. The transcript is what the person said and there is no interpretation at this point, so I would argue that it is not the best use of the participant's goodwill or the researcher's time. I believe it is far more useful to return later in the analysis to check the interpretation of the data to see whether the findings resonate with the person's perspective.

We did not use member checking in the Alone in a Crowd study, but we did present preliminary findings at conferences and workshops with groups of older people and service providers in each State. We also had a National Advisory Panel made up of key people from around the country who met regularly by teleconference, and we presented our findings to the panel for comment. A very valuable member of that group was from an advocacy group for older people, and their representative always gave us thoughtful and challenging feedback. Having a reference group comprising major stakeholders is a useful strategy for rigor and for guidance about broader issues in relation to the topic, networking, and ideas for dissemination strategies.

Ethical approval for this study was obtained from two university ethics committees and from each of the industry partner organizations. We paid particular attention to the issue of participants being free to make up their own minds about volunteering to participate and not feeling obliged given the pre-existing and ongoing nature of the relationship between residents or service users and the organization or workers and their employer. As we were collecting data in participants' homes and in rural locations, we also considered researcher safety. Data collectors wore name badges identifying them as coming from a university, carried a mobile phone, and someone knew where they were going and when they were expected to return.

Critiquing qualitative descriptive studies

While a generic approach to qualitative research with no alignment to a particular theoretical orientation is useful and appealing, it does pose some challenges for developing guidelines for critiquing qualitative descriptive studies. The questions I have developed (refer to Textbox 3.4) relate to qualitative descriptive studies that use a thematic analysis rather than content analysis.

Textbox 3.4　Critiquing qualitative descriptive studies – questions to ask

1　Has the *design* been chosen for an *exploratory, descriptive* study?
2　Does the research question fit with a *generic approach* that is not aligned to a particular theoretical orientation?
3　Are *methodological decisions* around sampling, recruitment, data collection, and rigor described in detail?
4　Are the steps used in *analysis described in detail*?
5　Do the findings presented show *interpretation and abstraction* without losing sight of the data?
6　Does the author make explicit how the *findings contribute to knowledge*?

Application to occupational science

On reviewing literature within occupational science, it appears that loneliness has received scant attention from an occupational perspective. Since completion of the larger Alone in a Crowd study, I have conducted a secondary analysis of the interview data extracting any sections of text that related to occupation and occupational engagement. That is, anything that the participants said about doing activities or the lack of activity. A similar thematic analysis process to that described earlier in this chapter was conducted on the subset of data resulting in the themes 'keeping active and engaged' and 'social connections'. The themes revealed that the older people understood loneliness in terms of not having meaningful occupations and mediated loneliness by engaging in occupations.

There is a need to engage with others in occupations that satisfy social needs and lead to a sense of belonging to the wider community. Engaging in meaningful occupations gives older people an opportunity to connect with others with shared interests which provides opportunity for forging deeper connections and friendship. The other connection mediated through engaging in occupation is to an occupational community. Having a meaningful occupation to engage in also provides a broad range of activities outside of the actual occupation, such as reading about it in magazines or on the Internet, shopping for clothing or tools associated with the occupation, or reminiscing about special times of engagement. Additionally, engaging in meaningful occupations when on one's own enables older people to feel satisfied and not feel lonely. The sense of connection to others appears to pervade the occupational engagement even when others are not physically present. The findings from this study contribute to knowledge about the interaction between occupational engagement and health and well-being.

From the Alone in a Crowd study, we know that social isolation and loneliness are different but closely related. Studying the experience of solitude rather than loneliness could potentially extend occupational science knowledge and make a useful contribution by gaining an understanding of how people meaningfully occupy their time when alone.

Application to occupational therapy

Given the new understandings about the role of occupation and engagement in occupation in how loneliness is understood and mediated, and the significant effects on health and well-being from being lonely, occupational therapists could take a more active role in enabling older people to prevent loneliness or to self-manage.

Knowing about the private dimension of loneliness and how stigmatized it is requires a sensitivity from occupational therapists to provide opportunities for clients to reveal loneliness. Given that loneliness is understood in terms of lack of meaningful occupation, we can use that as a clue when interviewing clients. An older person might say, well I used to do xx and I used to do xx, which should be a signal to the occupational therapist that engagement in meaningful occupations has altered and then can be followed up with a direct question about the experience of loneliness. Clients may need assistance to enable them to re-engage with meaningful occupations or to modify or replace occupations that are no longer within their capacity.

The adjustment dimension has an obvious fit with occupational therapy practice. Occupational therapists commonly work with clients following significant health events such as a stroke. While it might be common practice for occupational therapists to work with older people at times of major adjustment and adaptation, it is less likely that the issue of loneliness comes to the fore. Occupational therapists could make a significant difference for clients' well-being by bringing the issues of loneliness into sharper focus.

Furthermore, occupational therapists have an important role to play in preventing loneliness for older people. We know that there are times when older people are more vulnerable to loneliness such as after a significant health event, loss of a spouse or loss of a relationship, and when they relocate geographically. Prevention can occur at the individual, group, community or population level. For example, an occupational therapist might work with an individual who has become deconditioned through long-term hospitalization re-engage in occupations through a graded program. They might also connect that person to an appropriate community group. Using a community development approach occupational therapists could connect older people with like interests in the community or perhaps develop a website which educates and empowers older people and the wider community about loneliness and how to address or prevent it. As long as we only work at the individual or group level, the potential outcomes will be limited by the private nature and stigma of loneliness; therefore, we need to address loneliness at a population level as well, in partnership with older people.

Qualitative descriptive studies offer great potential for occupational therapy research without the need to understand an underlying theoretical orientation. They are particularly useful for evaluating client's and stakeholder's views on a program or service or a topic, and the findings can be used to inform quality improvements, more client-focused services, and better targeted services. The findings from qualitative descriptive studies are also readily conveyed by occupational therapists to clients or other team members without them requiring an understanding of a theoretical orientation in order to comprehend the findings.

Personal reflections

A descriptive qualitative approach was a good fit for a large study with multiple researchers. At times it was a challenge to reach consensus so that all researchers felt heard and valued, but that challenge related more to working across disciplines and geographical locations and time zones rather than the approach to the research.

I have conducted other studies using a descriptive qualitative approach and supervised numerous student projects. Having used grounded theory for my PhD and in my professional life having a strong attraction to processes I would say that I approach a descriptive qualitative design from a grounded, emergent, and social constructivist perspective. So while I might claim no particular alignment with a theoretical orientation for descriptive qualitative I think that my view of the world as socially constructed influences my teaching and research without me being consciously aware of that. My preference in data analysis is always, 'let's see what is in the data'; what emerges from analysis, rather than imposing a coding framework which could be an appropriate way to do the analysis. The key difference here is that the aim is to build a rich description rather than a theory.

I like the open generic nature of this approach. It lends itself to many of the research questions that I am interested in which are about gaining the perspective of various client groups as their view is often absent from the research literature. The outcome is a rich description of another's perspective. There is an appeal in revealing findings that might have been anticipated and that confirm what is already 'known' but there is scant evidence for. More importantly, I love how the 'taken for granted' or the unknown is revealed, as that is where the very special contribution to knowledge or practice lies. The private dimension of loneliness is a very good example of revealing the unknown or 'taken for granted', and I contend that it makes an important contribution to knowledge.

Summary

In this chapter, I have described the most generic methodology within qualitative research designs. I have drawn on the Alone in a Crowd study of older people and loneliness to show how a qualitative descriptive methodology can be utilized. In drawing on that experience, one of the features of this chapter has been to show how the methodology can be applied in a large project which attracted nationally competitive funding with attention paid to rigor. Just because the methodology is generic and not aligned to any particular theoretical orientation, it does not mean that it is second rate or less serious than other methodologies. Indeed, as was the case with the loneliness study, seeking the perspective of the end user of services, the taken for granted can be revealed providing direction for program and policy development and further research. Therein lies a great beauty which can equally apply to smaller scale studies conducted by a single researcher or a small team.

In the title of this chapter I called on a line from a song from a well-known musical, *The Sound of Music*, "Let's start at the very beginning, a very good place to start". At the conclusion of this chapter, I hesitate to draw it to a close but reiterate that qualitative descriptive work is a very good place to start for conducting research that will contribute to occupational science and inform occupational therapy practice.

References

Australian Bureau of Statistics. (2009). *Australian social trends 4102.0*. Retrieved from http://www.abs.gov.au/AUSSTATS/abs@.nsf/Lookup/4102.0Main+Features10March%202009

Creswell, J. (2007). *Qualitative inquiry and research design. Choosing among five approaches* (2nd ed.). Thousand Oaks, CA: Sage.

Davidson, C. (2009). Transcription: Imperatives for qualitative research. *International Journal of Qualitative Methods, 8*(2), 1–52.

Denzin, N. K., & Lincoln, Y. S. (2005). Introduction: The discipline and practice of qualitative research. In N. K. Denzin & Y. S. Lincoln (Eds.), *The SAGE handbook of qualitative research* (3rd ed., pp. 1–32). Thousand Oaks, CA: Sage

Gillham, B. (2000). *The research interview*. London, UK: Continuum.

Guba, E. G., & Lincoln, Y. S. (2005). Paradigmatic controversies, contradictions, and emerging confluences. In N. K. Denzin & Y. S. Lincoln (Eds.), *The SAGE handbook of qualitative research* (3rd ed., pp. 163–188). Thousand Oaks, CA: Sage.

Holmqvist, K., Kamwendo, K., & Ivasrsson, A.-B. (2009). Occupational therapists' descriptions of their work with persons suffering from cognitive impairment following acquired brain injury. *Scandinavian Journal of Occupational Therapy, 16*, 13–24

Kibele, A., & Llorens, L. A. (1989). Going to the source: The use of qualitative methodology in a study of the needs of adults with cerebral palsy. *Occupational Therapy in Health Care, 6*(2/3), 27–40.

Koome, F., Hocking, C., & Sutton, D. (2012). Why routines matter: The nature and meaning of family routines in the context of adolescent mental illness. *Journal of Occupational Science, 19*(4), 312–325

Kosma, A., Bryant, W., & Wilson, L. (2013). Drawing on Wilcock: An investigation of the impact of her published work on occupational therapy practice and research. *British Journal of Occupational Therapy, 76*(4), 179–185.

Liamputtong, P. (Ed.). (2013). *Research methods in health: Foundations for evidence-based practice* (2nd ed.). Melbourne, Australia: Oxford University Press.

Merrill, S. C. (1985). Qualitative methods in occupational therapy research: An application. *Occupational Therapy Journal of Research, 5*(4), 209–222.

Mishler, E. G. (1986). *Research interviewing. Context and narrative.* Cambridge: Harvard University Press.

Murray, C., & Lawry, J. (2011). Maintenance of professional currency: Perceptions of occupational therapists. *Australian Occupational Therapy Journal, 58*(4), 261–269.

Neergaard, M. A., Olesen, F., Andersen, R. S., & Sondergaard, J. (2009). Qualitative description – The poor cousin of health research? *BMC Medical Research Methodology, 9*(52), 1–5.

O'Connor, A., Cahill, M., & McKay, E. A. (2012). Revisiting 1:1 and 2:1 clinical placement models: Student and clinical educator perspectives. *Australian Occupational Therapy Journal, 59*, 276–283.

Patton, M. Q. (2002). *Qualitative research and evaluation methods* (3rd ed.). Thousand Oaks, CA: Sage.

Sandelowski, M. (2000). Whatever happened to qualitative description? *Research in Nursing and Health, 23*, 334–340.

Sandelowski, M. (2010). What's in a name? Qualitative description revisited. *Research in Nursing and Health, 33*, 77–84.

Stanley, M., Moyle, W., Ballantyne, A., Jaworski, K., Corlis, M., Oxlade, D., . . . Young, B. (2010). 'Nowadays you don't even see your neighbours': Loneliness in the everyday lives of older Australians. *Health and Social Care in the Community, 18*(4), 407–417.

Thorne, S., & Derbyshire, P. (2005). Land mines in the field: A modest proposal for improving the craft of qualitative research. *Qualitative Health Research, 15*, 1105–1113.

Thorne, S., Kirkham, S., & O'Flynn-Magee, K. (2004). The analytic challenge in interpretive descriptive description. *International Journal of Qualitative Methods, 3*(1), 1–11.

Further reading

Schwandt, T. A. (2007). *The SAGE dictionary of qualitative inquiry* (3rd ed.). Thousand Oaks, CA: Sage.

Patton, M. Q. (2002). *Qualitative research and evaluation methods* (3rd ed.). Thousand Oaks, CA: Sage.

4 Grounded theory

Uncovering a world of process

Shoba Nayar

Perseverance. Patience. Passion. If these are words that you identify with as a researcher, then grounded theory may be a good methodological fit for you. However, using grounded theory methodology for any study is a journey in itself; so even if you are unsure whether these words reflect you, I invite you to consider the world of grounded theory. In this chapter I draw on my study of the occupational processes of Indian immigrant women settling in New Zealand to demonstrate the application and benefits of using grounded theory methodology for occupation-focused research.

Described as an "empirical approach to the study of social life through qualitative research and distinctive approaches to data analysis" (Clarke, 2005, p. xxi), grounded theory is capable of exploring and understanding social processes that occur within society. Introduced by sociologists Barney Glaser and Anselm Strauss (1967), grounded theory resonated with social scientists who were interested in generating new theory as opposed to testing existing theory in what was otherwise a positivist environment (Birks & Mills, 2011).

Nursing scholars, in particular, have embraced this methodology with many grounded theory studies addressing aspects of the provision of nursing care. Although it has been used to a lesser extent in occupation-focused research, Stanley and Cheek (2003) have advocated for grounded theory as a methodological approach to study the "use of occupations to enhance health and wellbeing" (p. 143). Examples of grounded theory studies used in occupational science and occupational therapy address topics such as the well-being of older people (Stanley, 2006), the settlement experiences of immigrants (Kim & Nayar, 2012; Nayar, Hocking, & Giddings, 2012) and the inter-professional collaborative learning process of occupational therapy and other allied health students (Howell, 2009). However, there is still plenty of scope for occupation-focused grounded theory studies.

Background

In time, grounded theory methodology has evolved to encompass different nuances and approaches. These iterations have been led by many former students of Glaser and Strauss, from their time teaching at the University of California,

San Francisco. For instance, Charmaz (2006), a former occupational therapist, has been one proponent advancing the development of grounded theory, along with contemporaries such as Clarke (2005), Bowers (Bowers & Schatzman, 2009), and Corbin (2009), who together have become known as the second generation of grounded theorists. Despite the variations, the ultimate aim of grounded theory methodology is still apparent, that is, to discover and explain the underlying social processes shaping interaction and human behavior. It is this aim that underpins the resonance between grounded theory and occupation-focused research.

There are multiple opportunities for the use of grounded theory in occupation-centered studies, reflecting that many social processes involve engagement in occupation. As a discipline, occupational science seeks to influence society, while keeping the notion of occupation central to understanding the everyday experiences of people's lives. Implicit in the 'everyday experiences' is the notion of 'process' or doing as it unfolds over time. From this perspective, grounded theory methodology has much to offer for extending our understandings of people's occupational engagement.

The work that occupational therapists are engaged in is, primarily, process driven. Whether it is assisting clients in their recovery from mental illness or stroke, transitioning from unemployment to paid work or encouraging children in play, all are examples of occupation-rich processes. Furthermore, the work of occupational therapists shifts within and across time, similar to the practice of grounded theory methods which involves the interplay between data collection and data analysis (Charmaz, 2006). Concurrent data collection and analysis means that the researcher is constantly moving from the present to consider what has happened in the past and what may happen in the future. A social process is dynamic, much the same as engagement in occupation. Both contain movement and develop as new pieces of data/understanding become apparent or previously analyzed data take on new meaning. The ultimate act of grounded theory is, therefore, to uncover the social processes individuals use in response to a particular phenomenon that includes elements of the past, present, and future.

Epistemology

The variations within grounded theory, such as classic (Glaser, 1992) or constructivist (Charmaz, 2006) approaches, make defining the theoretical orientation difficult. Glaser, for instance, would argue that grounded theory has no philosophical underpinning. However, given the focus of grounded theory research on social processes which occur over time, symbolic interactionism, which focuses on the ways by which individuals interact, interpret, and make meaning of their world (Blumer, 1969), is often considered the underpinning theoretical perspective.

From a symbolic interactionist perspective, the social and political context within which the person operates is central in shaping personal beliefs, values, thoughts, and actions. That is, the environment within which we reside constructs the self and subsequent actions. The self in symbolic interactionism is a duality comprising both a *me* and an *I*. The thinking part of us is directed by the *I*. The *I* processes information and makes a decision about how the interaction will proceed. The actual act – or interaction – is led by the *me* aspect of self which is the interactor between the self and society. Thus, it is the *I* which interprets and contributes meaning to an event, and it is the *me* which subsequently acts (Bowers, 1988). The environment with its variety of conditions and contexts elicits change in people and shapes their actions in order to make sense of the world. Reality is therefore a social construct – hence the synergy between symbolic interactionism and grounded theory. Ultimately, no matter how the researcher positions himself or herself, clearly articulating the theoretical orientation is pivotal for laying the foundations of a rigorous study as it will guide data analysis and presentation of findings.

Defining the topic

Grounded theory is particularly useful in areas where little is known about the phenomenon of interest or where there are few existing theories to explain an individual's or group's behavior. My interest in the settlement processes of Indian immigrants living in New Zealand stemmed from my experiences as an occupational therapist working with immigrants in a mental health service and self-identification as an Indian immigrant woman who has witnessed and experienced the challenges of settling in a new environment. Having identified my topic, I reviewed the relevant occupational therapy, occupational science, and migration literature. There was literature regarding psychological well-being, employment, and parenting; however, it appeared that the everyday occupations, such as shopping, socializing, and driving, had not been considered as the central concern for many of the studies. My study therefore aimed to address the gap in the literature and to generate a theory about settlement based on the experiences of Indian women who had migrated to New Zealand.

There is much debate about the place of a literature review in a grounded theory study. Glaser (1978) contended that the researcher should not look at the literature prior to undertaking the study as it may influence the researcher's assumptions and analysis of data. However, funding bodies, ethics committees, and academic institutions often require some review of the literature when writing research proposals. Thus, an initial literature review can be done with the purpose of ascertaining the gap to be studied. Literature is then incorporated as data are collected and analyzed (as discussed later in this chapter).

Having decided on a topic, the next step is to develop the research question. In a grounded theory study, the research question commonly starts with 'how'; for example, 'how do Indian immigrant women settle in New Zealand?' or 'how do occupational therapists use evidence to inform practice?' In some instances, questions may begin with 'what'; for example, 'what happens when occupational therapists undertake postgraduate study?' The key to constructing a grounded theory question is to focus on process.

Recruitment and sampling

In a grounded theory study, recruitment follows techniques common to many qualitative studies, for example, the use of flyers, word of mouth or intermediaries.

However, sampling in grounded theory occurs across two stages: (1) purposive and (2) theoretical. A hallmark of grounded theory is the concurrent data collection and analysis; thus, initially a purposive sample of people who fit the inclusion criteria are sought. To be eligible for inclusion in my study, participants were required to have immigrated to New Zealand between the years of 1980 and 2006. This criterion was important for capturing the complexity of the settlement process as it unfolds over time. I was keen to see whether there might be similarities in the process for women who had emigrated 20 years ago compared with women who had been in the country for only 4 years. A rise in the numbers of Indian immigrants arriving each year has fuelled the development of resources to meet the needs of this population. For instance, in the early 1980s in New Zealand, it was rare to find shops selling Indian spices and groceries. These days, Indian grocery stores are relatively accessible, particularly in the larger cities; therefore, I assumed that the process of doing things 20 years ago would be different from how things are done today.

In sampling participants for a grounded theory study, maximum variation adds depth to the evolving theory. Thus, in addition to the time resident in New Zealand, I also considered location and recruited participants from two large cities with established Indian populations and two smaller cities with comparably fewer Indian immigrants. Initially, four participants were purposively sampled and formed a diverse group in terms of age, length of time since migration, who they emigrated with, and the number of people known in New Zealand before emigrating. As analysis progresses, theoretical sampling is used to seek participants who can best provide answers to enhance understandings of emerging concepts.

Theoretical sampling

Theoretical sampling guides decision making and assists with seeking participants who can provide data that will clarify dimensions of emerging categories; thus participants are selected as research progresses rather than being pre-determined. According to Strauss and Corbin (1998), theoretical sampling is key to grounded theory methodology as it enables the researcher to obtain a participant population that will maximize opportunities to compare events and "bring about greatest theoretical return" (p. 202). For example, the first five participants had all immigrated with their families. As such, their stories about settling in New Zealand were often influenced by what they needed to do for their children. Therefore, in recruiting the sixth participant, I deliberately sought someone who had immigrated by herself to see how her story of creating a place in New Zealand was similar or different to the processes of women with families.

Ideally, sampling and collection of data continues until theoretical saturation is reached. That is, the researcher becomes aware that no new data relating to the categories are emerging, that relationships between categories have been fully developed and all aspects of the theory are substantiated. However, it needs to be acknowledged that project limitations such as time frames and finances may prevent this from happening.

Data collection methods

A range of data can be used in a grounded theory study including documents, participant observations, and/or in-depth interviews – either individual or focus groups. If using focus groups, it is recommended that these occur at the start of the study in determining what the central concern is for participants. Once theoretical sampling commences, data collection should take the form of individual interviews. In my study, in-depth interviews were the primary source of data and participant observations formed a secondary source of data. Both are suitable for studies exploring occupation which can best be understood through narratives of occupation or observation of people engaging in occupation. Additionally, I collected basic demographic data such as age, who participants immigrated with, and year of arrival.

Individual in-depth interviews

Interviews were held in the participants' home or workplace. The initial four interviews opened with a request statement, 'Tell me about doing things differently in New Zealand'. As an opening prompt, I soon realized that it did not naturally lead particpants to talking about their experiences of immigrating; what went well, what they struggled with or what they would do differently if they emigrated again. The question was too focussed on eliciting stories of occupation as opposed to leaving room for participants to talk abut what mattered most to them in their process of settling in New Zealand. Thus, I began the next set of interviews with the opening request statement 'Tell me about migrating to New Zealand'.

From this initial statement, I then asked clarifying questions to elicit further information. As data analyses progressed, I continued to open with the same question to warm participants up to the focus of the research; after which, in line with theoretical sampling, I began asking specific questions to assist with developing dimensions of emerging concepts, arising during the course of analysis (Bowers, 1988) (see Textbox 4.1).

Textbox 4.1   Clarifying questions

In an interview with Anaia, I sought to clarify her comments on the learning she had done as a teacher in New Zealand:

A: Though we teach, in India it's a little different, here it's more practical. Everything the planning and, it's very nice, very well organized but it's good, so I learned it.

***Shoba:* So the learning that went on, how did that learning occur?**

As data analysis progresses, I had conceptualized that there was a relationship between participants' feelings of 'acceptance' and their feelings of 'being settled'. To find out more about this relationship I asked Neha:

(continued)

(continued)

Shoba:	**If you don't feel accepted here in New Zealand, or feel you don't belong in this country, is it possible for you to feel settled here?**
N:	A very interesting question. I feel quite, I'm settled into the ways, the daily life of New Zealand, I can go through a day and come back okay but, I don't feel happy . . . So, I think I'm settled into daily life, so that's something that obviously you have to, you have to be settled because of your child, you have to at least give a semblance of being settled to your child. But deep down happy, no because, I'm just constantly juggling, I'm juggling too much to be happy.

Participant observations

Field observations of participants engaging in occupations as part of living in New Zealand, such as going to work, attending social events, or preparing meals, were used to supplement information elicited during individual interviews. For example, in an interview one of the participants talked about the difficulty she experienced socializing with her colleagues at work. Following the interview, I arranged to spend the day with her at her workplace. As I sat observing the environment, it became clear that the difficulty with socializing was a result of physical and institutional barriers. The desks were arranged in groups of four with high partitions blocking her view of the other desks, so that once seated, she was unable to interact with her fellow colleagues. Further, she was told by her manager, at the beginning of her shift, when to take her breaks; thus, preventing her from spontaneously joining colleagues for lunch. Without the opportunity to observe her work setting, I may have interpreted the information from her interview as a lack of social inclusion by work colleagues due to cultural differences.

Memoing

Memoing is a central process in grounded theory and a technique used by researchers to record their thinking processes concerning the products of analysis or directions for further analysis (Richards, 2005). For the grounded theory researcher, memoing is a central process (Strauss, 1987). Glaser (1978) argued that "the bedrock of theory generation, its true product is the writing of theoretical memos. If the analyst skips this stage by going directly from coding to sorting or to writing – he is *not* doing grounded theory" (p. 83). Memos may involve drawing models and/or diagrams that designate relationships between categories to help progress theory or may be written reflections on the research process as it unfolds. In whatever manner memos are constructed, they are meant to be "analytical and conceptual rather than descriptive" (Strauss & Corbin, 1998, p. 217). In Textbox 4.2, I include an example of memoing from my study.

Textbox 4.2   Example of memoing

I utilized memos in various ways throughout the process: to generate questions about the data I had collected, capture thoughts regarding the development of concepts and to map out relationship between concepts. The following memo written during data analysis assisted with making decisions regarding ongoing data collection and theoretical sampling and questioning:

> 12.06.07: In the interview today A talked about feeling different or being different until she gets to 'that stage'. What does she mean by 'that stage'? What does 'that stage' look like? When will she know if she has reached 'that stage'? Do other women have a sense of needing to reach a 'stage' before they feel completely accepted and no longer different? Is a stage something fixed, like a stage on which people perform, or is it moveable? Do people return to the stage at different times, in different contexts? Perhaps a question I might ask in the next interview is *Do you think there is a stage that you need to reach before you no longer feel different? If so how would you describe that stage?*

The participant in the above example had been in the country for 5 years and seemed to have this notion of a 'stage' that she had not yet reached. Analyzing the data from this interview, 'stage' felt like a significant concept that warranted further exploration. I wondered whether 'stages' were indicative of a linear process and if so, was this an accurate reflection of the process immigrants go through when settling in a new country? In considering how stages might develop or how many stages there are, I sought to talk with a woman who had lived in New Zealand for a longer period of time and who might be able to offer more insights into the concept of 'stages'.

Data analysis

Analysis commences simultaneously with the start of data collection. Thus grounded theory analysis is an iterative process of analysis, returning to the field for more data and back to analysis. The process of grounded theory analysis tends to be more structured than other qualitative approaches. Data are read and analyzed word by word, line by line, as part of a coding process. These initial codes are then grouped as 'categories' or 'concepts', which refer to the context, strategies, and conditions under which the social process unfolds. Ultimately, each of these categories is linked to a central process or core category.

The coding process

I began the coding process using open coding or substantive coding, which is the first stage of analysis (Glaser & Strauss, 1967) and requires data to be "broken down into discrete parts, closely examined, and compared for similarities and differences" (Strauss & Corbin, 1998, p. 102). Coding is a process of organizing data through sorting and labeling. To begin coding, I examined the interview transcripts line-by-line to identify concepts that represent phenomena. During this examination, labels were given to sentences or phrases that captured the meaning of the phenomenon. These labels became codes that describe the concepts which arise directly from words or phrases in the data, also known as 'in-vivo codes'. For example the line of transcript, "I had to negotiate with the children, it was always like you brought us here, so you'd better help out" (Jean) was coded 'negotiating with children'.

One aim in generating codes is to name them using action words. For example, initial coding revealed the concept 'building a platform'; a platform being a foundation that the women could use to assist with settling in New Zealand. In generating a code for this concept, I used the word 'Platforming'. Glaser (1978) termed this approach to analysis 'gerund grounded theory', and using this process often helps the researcher to consider what it is that participants are doing, which then facilitates the constant comparison of experiences.

Constant comparative analysis

Data collected in a grounded theory study are analyzed using constant comparative analysis, a hallmark of grounded theory studies. Using this method, I worked my way through the interview transcripts comparing initial codes and looking for similarities and points of difference in my analysis. According to Hutchinson (1986), this type of interplay between the data allows for a proposed theory that is "molecular in structure rather than causal or linear" (p. 122). Constant comparative analysis is used within grounded theory studies to aid with theoretical decision making and can be used to assist with preparing and asking questions in later interviews to deepen understanding of emerging concepts.

My initial interviews were conducted with participants living in Auckland and Hamilton, cities which have a comparatively larger Indian population to the rest of the country. In these interviews, I discovered that having access to resources connected to India, such as Indian grocery products, places of worship, other Indian people, meant that the women could effectively maintain connection with their country of origin while establishing a new home for themselves and their families in New Zealand. When there was greater access to Indian resources, the women had more choices in terms of whether they engaged with Indian practices or adopted New Zealand ways of performing occupations. I began to compare interviews, looking for instances of where participants talked about engaging in Indian activities versus New Zealand activities and what they had available to them that facilitated their choice in any given situation. Furthermore, as I engaged in theoretical sampling, I began to ask theoretical questions related to the role of the Indian community and how the Indian community facilitated settlement.

Given my findings above, in that having access to Indian resources strengthened the women's ability to stay connected to their culture, I was keen to get another perspective. Therefore, I attempted to recruit women from smaller cities and more rural parts of the country. Despite the use of personal contacts this proved a challenging task; however, I was able to locate participants in the city of Hastings. What emerged from these interviews and theoretical questioning was that in a city where there was a significantly smaller Indian population and limited access to Indian resources, there was less willingness to be seen performing culturally mediated occupations out in public, community spaces. Engaging in constant comparative analysis allowed me to generate theoretical questions to further the development of specific concepts, such as 'Working with Indian Ways' and thus deepen the analysis.

As data analysis proceeded, the use of constant comparative analysis both guided further interviews and what to look for in the data and took me back to the literature. In grounded theory, literature becomes part of the method by which the theory is compared, contrasted, sorted, and expanded (Glaser, 1992). Thus, as pertinent concepts developed, I returned to the literature. For instance, at this point in my analysis, I was beginning to establish a concept around 'place' and the importance of 'creating a space in which to live'. With this framework, I read about notions of place and environment and how these are constructed.

Developing the theory

It is important to carefully consider which variant of grounded theory will be used for a grounded theory study. Indeed, as one strategy for rigor, researchers are advised to make explicit which version of grounded theory they are using and to describe and justify any deviation from the chosen approach (Cutcliffe, 2000). While all approaches follow the methods of open coding and constant comparative analysis, the process of developing codes into abstract categories and eventually a theory to explain the social process can differ. For example, Glaser (1978) described a process of selective coding followed by theoretical coding. Strauss and Corbin (1998) developed a conditional matrix, a more structured approach for the novice grounded theorist. I chose to follow Schatzman (1991; Bowers & Schatzman, 2009) and his variant of dimensional analysis.

The dimensional matrix provides a framework for the ordering and conceptualizing of data (Schatzman, 1991). Within the dimensional matrix are the elements which reflect the "complexity of a phenomenon by noting its attributes, context, processes and meaning" (Kools, McCarthy, Durham, & Robrecht, 1996, p. 315). When using the matrix to organize data, Schatzman proposed that every dimension needs to be given an opportunity to act as perspective or context. By changing the perspective and/or the context, the opportunity arises for the whole process to change. Figure 4.1 shows a dimensional matrix with all the categories developed in the study. In this stage of analysis, I created multiple matrices, shifting categories to different places, for example, moving Keeping Past and Present from a strategy to a perspective as a means of understanding how that shift would change the placement of other categories and subsequently the overall relationship.

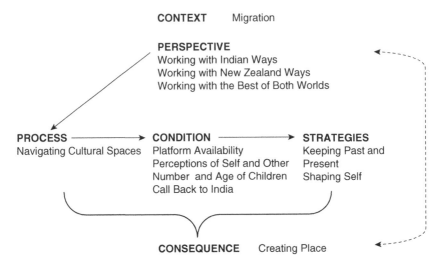

Figure 4.1 Dimensional matrix over-viewing categories

Using the dimensional matrices to plot different relationships among the salient dimensions that had arisen through the analytic process enabled me to create a coherent whole identifying the relationships between my concepts and lifting the level of abstraction to a substantive theory of the process Indian immigrant women engage in when creating a place in a new environment.

Findings: core category

A fully developed grounded theory study must have a core category. The core category emerges from the data and has the explanatory power to pull together the theory (Glaser, 1978) – linking categories and explaining any variation in the process. It is the core category which captures the social process and human interactions that occur in the phenomenon.

Navigating Cultural Spaces is the core process in this substantive theory and emerges as a result of the women's efforts to move between their known ways of doing everyday tasks and new occupations for the purpose of Creating a Place for themselves and their families as Indian immigrants living in New Zealand. Occupations occur in different environments, involve a variety of skills, engage individuals and collective groups, and are performed consciously and unconsciously. Within this process, the women were constantly navigating the need to keep themselves safe, knowing their capabilities, and making the most of opportunities for exploring new ways of doing everyday occupations. By engaging in occupations, the women *Navigated Cultural Spaces* either by themselves or with others, interacting with their environment, and engaging in multiple ways of performing occupations, thus, moving between the cultural boundaries for the purpose of settling in New Zealand.

There were times when *Navigating Cultural Spaces* meant the women sought safety in performing occupations that were familiar and representative of their culture before venturing out to try something new – a perspective of Working with Indian Ways. Alternatively, there were times when the women experimented with trying to do things influenced by the New Zealand culture – Working with New Zealand Ways – thus acquiring new skills and resources before perhaps returning to what was familiar. Ultimately, the desire for many women was to find a way of blending the components of different cultures within their daily occupations – Working with the Best of Both Worlds – for the purpose of Creating a Place in New Zealand.

The women moved between the different Ways of Working depending on certain conditions. For instance, if they had children of a young age they were more likely to engage in occupations reflective of Indian Ways. When they had a positive perception of others and felt that they would be welcomed, then they would more readily try engaging in occupations that reflected the New Zealand culture. Navigating Cultural Spaces also required the women to use certain strategies, such as bringing resources from India, for example, particular cooking supplies – an act of Keeping Past and Present – in order to continue Working with Indian Ways. In this way, the process of settling in New Zealand for Indian immigrant women involved complex navigation (Figure 4.2).

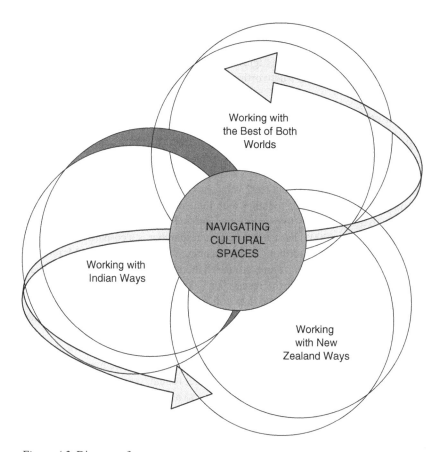

Figure 4.2 Diagram of core category

Data management

Qualitative studies can generate large amounts of textual data. Therefore, before commencing analysis it is important to consider how data will be managed. I was introduced to NVivo by a colleague using the software for her own qualitative research. The benefit of using computer software is that it is a technical tool that can store large amounts of data and ideas, which can then be retrieved quickly and efficiently (Richards, 2005). For instance, if I noticed a repetitive pattern, I was able to run a word search and see how often, and across how many interviews, that notion occurred. The 'best of both worlds' was a phrase I had heard spoken by many of my participants. When I ran a search for this phrase it appeared in 19 out of the 25 interviews; thus, I could conclude that it was an important concept. As a tool NVivo does not analyze the data; rather, it is designed to assist the researcher with organization of data. In the initial stages of grounded theory analysis where a number of codes were generated, I found the programming too cumbersome to be able to hold, sort, and organize all my codes. I also found myself getting frustrated at not being able to see all the data at once on the screen. Thus I returned to my preferred style of 'pencil and paper' for doing analytic work.

Initially, I coded by hand directly on the transcript. I then cut up subsequent transcripts, placing quotes against codes, and clustering to form categories. I also began drawing diagrams as a way of visually playing with the data to develop the relationships between categories (Figure 4.1). These diagrams formed part of the audit trail contributing to the trustworthiness of the findings.

Rigor and ethics

Good grounded theory is not about imposing pre-existing theories; rather it is about generating theory that is grounded in the data. Yet, researchers are never completely impartial. As humans, researchers bring their past experiences, knowledge, and values to the process. Indeed, Glaser (1992) suggested that it is the researcher's professional and personal experience together with their in-depth knowledge of the data that gives them the sensitivity to generate categories. Further, from a constructionist perspective, Charmaz (2006) has argued that the researcher is a co-participant in the study whose experiences contribute to the phenomena being explored. 'Memoing' is the primary technique for rigor in a grounded theory study. As written records of analysis, memos make explicit the researcher's decisions, and assist with exploring issues of concern throughout the data collection and analysis process. Keeping detailed audit trails and making transparent the research process throughout the study write up strengthens the position of the grounded theory researcher.

In addition to memoing, appraisers of qualitative rigor often look for the use of member checking and triangulation; however, these are not mandatory in a grounded theory study. The researcher uses theoretical sampling to determine who to talk to next or which interview questions to ask to expand on the emergent theory rather than using member checking. When done well, participants will be able to identify their journey in the grounded theory, and this is testament to the rigor of the study.

From an ethical perspective, theoretical sampling may present challenges. For instance, a number of participants may be recruited, yet not all may be sampled to take part in the study due to the need to follow the research process and interview participants who can best speak of emerging theoretical concepts. If potential participants are recruited but not interviewed for the study, it is important, at a minimum, to offer them a summary of the research findings in recognition of their willingness to be involved.

Critiquing grounded theory studies

Many published studies using grounded theory methodology do not result in the development of a theory. More commonly, these articles use grounded theory methods of analysis, for example, Strauss and Corbin's (1998) three stages of open, axial, and selective coding, in the framework of a qualitative descriptive study to develop themes. Thus, the findings often lack a core category and are not reflective of a social process – two key elements of a grounded theory study. Hence, it is important to ask some critical questions when reading grounded theory studies (Textbox 4.3).

Textbox 4.3   Critiquing grounded theory studies – questions to ask

1 Is the *epistemology* (symbolic interactionism or otherwise) clearly stated and justified?
2 Do the authors state what *variant of grounded theory* is being used?
3 Does the research question start with a *how* or *what*?
4 Is the research question *process* oriented?
5 Is there discussion of *theoretical sampling*?
6 Have the authors explained their method of *constant comparative analysis*?
7 Have the authors used *memos* as part of rigor?
8 Is there a *core category* presented?
9 Do the categories relate to each other and form a *coherent theory*?
10 Has the theory been *situated in current literature*?

Application to occupational science

What this current study has shown is that the things Indian immigrant women do in their daily lives and the occupational situations they encounter are dynamic events that either facilitate and enhance the experience of being in a new environment or challenge the process of settling and becoming part of the New Zealand context. Although it has long been acknowledged within occupational science that occupation is contextual, understandings of how occupation mediates person–place interactions, for particular social groups such as immigrants, have been limited.

This study revealed similarities in the participants' response to a new environment and how this shapes their occupational experiences. It also acknowledges that people are unique individuals, and therefore while on some levels there are similarities in the women's processes, the environment–occupation–person relationship is distinct for each individual. With increasing groups immigrating or gaining refugee status worldwide, there is a need for enhanced understanding of the central role that occupation has in mediating people's interaction with environment and their perception of self and well-being. Thus, the key conclusion or relevance to occupational science, as posited in this study, is the critical impact context has on immigrants' occupations and connections.

Application to occupational therapy

In a practice setting, clinical or otherwise, occupational therapists are likely to work with immigrant populations. This study identified that for many of the women having initial support from others helped with learning where to perform occupations, such as grocery shopping, and how to perform occupations, such as going to the doctor. This support came in either the practical form of having someone to do the occupation alongside them or in the form of instructions and being provided with the information needed to successfully complete the task. Thus, for therapists, study findings highlight the importance of 'doing with' clients in practice, rather than simply providing relevant information.

In addition to providing practical support, occupational therapists might consider establishing educational services in the form of groups. Developing support groups within the local community that new immigrants can attend and share their experiences of trying to do things in a new environment may be beneficial for assisting with the creation of an extended network of support, particularly for those immigrants who are in the country without family. These support groups might also provide a rich insight into the information immigrants need through the questions asked at such gatherings.

Finally, supporting immigrants to engage in a range of occupations that provide both comfort and safety and concurrently extend or challenge their abilities is important for living in a community with multiple cultures. Therapists may find the strategies developed as part of this grounded theory study useful in assisting immigrants with their daily occupations as part of the settlement process.

Personal reflections

As a person who likes playing with numbers as much as words, I was initially drawn to grounded theory as it appeared to be one of the more 'structured' qualitative methodologies with regard to analytic methods. I also tend to be someone who is interested, not so much, in the final outcome, but the pathways to that outcome. What decisions were made? When? By whom? What influenced those decisions? Asking those types of questions aligned with a grounded theory approach.

While grounded theory methods offer some structure, the methodology also requires creativity. One of the challenges has been to take the words of the participants and build something from the 'ground up' – a theory that is abstract enough to capture the social process, while still grounded in the data to reflect the variations that occur within participants' lives. In this process, I found having a critical group of other grounded theory researchers with whom I could discuss the evolving theory as an important part of my journey. Many times I thought I had my core category, only to find that when I presented it to a group of critical friends I was showered with questions that had me returning to the data. However, the satisfaction when the theory finally came together in that 'aha' moment was immense.

Finally, grounded theory has required discipline and at times sacrifices. Staying true to the methodology and the iterative process of analysis and data collection takes time, requires immersion in the process and analysis cannot be forced. Thus, having the support of mentors and critical friends is valuable.

Summary

Grounded theory is a recursive process; thus I return to the beginning of this chapter. Perseverance. Patience. Passion. Perseverance is needed to keep working with the data to develop a core category and a theory that coherently and robustly explains the social process. Patience is required for sitting in those times of 'not knowing' – where a potential theory lies but has not yet emerged. During these times, it is important to keep memoing every decision, question, and plan. Finally, a grounded theory study requires passion, a desire to understand the process, the journey toward reaching an outcome. When approached with these three values, grounded theory, as a qualitative methodology, has much to offer researchers in occupational science and occupational therapy who are interested in uncovering a world of process within which people engage in occupation.

References

Birks, M., & Mills, J. (2011). *Grounded theory a practical guide.* London, UK: Sage.

Blumer, H. (1969). *Symbolic interactionsim: Perspective and method.* London, UK: University of California Press.

Bowers, B. J. (1988). Grounded theory. In B. Sarter (Ed.), *Paths to knowledge: Innovative research methods for nursing* (pp. 33–59). New York, NY: National League for Nursing.

Bowers, B., & Schatzman, L. (2009). Dimensional analysis. In J. M. Morse, P. N. Stern, J. Corbin, B. Bowers, K. Charmaz, & A. E. Clarke (Eds.), *Developing grounded theory. The second generation* (pp. 90–132). Walnut Creek, CA: Left Coast Press.

Charmaz, K. (2006). *Constructing grounded theory: A practical guide through qualitative analysis.* Thousand Oaks, CA: Sage.

Clarke, A. E. (2005). *Situational analysis: Grounded theory after the postmodern turn.* Thousand Oaks, CA: Sage.

Corbin, J. (2009). Taking an analytic journey. In J. M. Morse, P. N. Stern, J. Corbin, B. Bowers, K. Charmaz, & A. E. Clarke (Eds.), *Developing grounded theory. The second generation* (pp. 35–54). Walnut Creek, CA: Left Coast Press.

Cutcliffe, J. (2000). Methodological issues in grounded theory. *Journal of Advanced Nursing, 31*(6), 1476–1484.

Glaser, B. G. (1978). *Theoretical sensitivity: Advances in the methodology of grounded theory.* Mill Valley, CA: Sociology Press.

Glaser, B. G. (1992). *Basics of grounded theory analysis.* Mill Valley, CA: Sociology Press.

Glaser, B. G., & Strauss, A. L. (1967). *The discovery of grounded theory: Strategies for qualitative research.* Chicago: Adeline De Gruyter.

Howell, D. (2009). Occupational therapy students in the process of interprofessional collaborative learning: A grounded theory study. *Journal of Interprofessional Care, 23*(1), 67–80. doi:10.1080/13561820802413281.

Hutchinson, S. (1986). Grounded theory. In P. Munhall & C. Oiler (Eds.), *Nursing research: A qualitative perspective* (pp. 111–130). New York, NY: National League for Nursing.

Kim, H., & Nayar, S. (2012). The experiences of Korean immigrants settling in New Zealand. In A. Sobrun-Maharaj, F. Rossen, S. Parackal, S. Nayar, E. Ho, D. Newcombe, . . . S. Ameratunga, (Eds.), *Social environment, migration and health. Proceedings of the Fifth International Asian and Ethnic Minority Health and Wellbeing Conference, June 27–28* (pp. 19–30). Auckland, New Zealand: University of Auckland.

Kools, S., McCarthy, M., Durham, R., & Robrecht, L. (1996). Dimensional analysis: Broadening the conception of grounded theory. *Qualitative Health Research, 6*(3), 312–330.

Nayar, S., Hocking, C., & Giddings, L. (2012). Using occupation to navigate cultural spaces: Indian immigrant women settling in New Zealand. *Journal of Occupational Science, 19*(1), 62–75. doi:10.1080/14427591.2011.602628.

Richards, L. (2005). *Handling qualitative data: A practical guide.* Thousand Oaks, CA: Sage.

Schatzman, L. (1991). Dimensional analysis: Notes on an alternative approach to the grounding of theory in qualitative research. In D. R. Maines (Ed.), *Social organization and social process* (pp. 303–314). New York, NY: Aldine De Gruyter.

Stanley, M. (2006). A grounded theory of the wellbeing of older people. In L. Finlay & C. Ballinger (Eds.), *Qualitative research for allied health professionals. challenging choices* (pp. 63–78). London, UK: John Wiley & Sons.

Stanley, M., & Cheek, J. (2003). Grounded theory: Exploiting the potential for occupational therapy. *British Journal of Occupational Therapy, 66*(4), 143–150.

Strauss, A. L. (1987). *Qualitative analysis for social scientists.* New York, NY: Cambridge University Press.

Strauss, A. L., & Corbin, J. (1998). *Basics of qualitative research: Techniques and procedures for developing grounded theory* (2nd ed.). Thousand Oaks, CA: Sage.

Further reading

Backman, K., & Kyngäs, H. A. (1999). Challenges of the grounded theory approach to a novice researcher. *Nursing and Health Science, 1*, 147–153.

Birks, M., Chapman, Y., & Francis, K. (2008). Memoing in qualitative research: Probing data and processes. *Journal of Research in Nursing, 13*(1), 68–75. doi:10.1177/174 4987107081254.

Bryant, A., & Charmaz, K. (2007). *The sage handbook of grounded theory.* London, UK: Sage.

Chentiz, W. C., & Swanson, J. M. (1986). *From practice to grounded theory: Qualitative research in nursing.* Menlo Park, CA: Addison-Wesley Publishing.

Website

http://www.groundedtheoryonline.com/

5   Doing (interpretive) phenomenology

Valerie Wright-St Clair

Thinking and writing, and writing and thinking, are defining ways of doing phenomenology. Being patient is an asset. You cannot make thinking come on demand; those 'aha' moments in understanding what the research text is saying will come through being immersed in, and staying engaged with, the data. Understanding the *meaning* of the phenomenon of interest is the phenomenologist's task. In this chapter, I focus on interpretive phenomenology, sometimes called hermeneutic or Heideggerian phenomenology, because it goes beyond rich descriptions of things, toward understanding. This distinction is important when exploring how a phenomenon appears, both as it is experienced by people and as it is interpreted by them. The seemingly complex language can be off-putting at first, but journey with me through this chapter and you will be rewarded by coming to see what makes interpretive phenomenology, interpretive phenomenology. Throughout the chapter I draw on an interpretive phenomenological study of older New Zealanders' experiences of being aged in their everyday. By the end of the chapter you will see what makes a study phenomenological in its nature and how it is suitable for occupation-focused research.

Background

Phenomenology is a philosophy and not a research methodology as such. It is a way of inquiry (Dreyfus, 1991); a way of thinking, of questioning, of writing, and of being a researcher. Therefore it is important for a phenomenological researcher to understand enough of the underpinning philosophy in order to interpret and apply it when designing and conducting an inquiry. Textbox 5.1 provides an overview of the research paradigms that phenomenology can be situated within and some of the associated philosophers (Pernecky & Jamal, 2010).

**Textbox 5.1   Situating phenomenology in the research
                 paradigms**

Husserl is widely acknowledged as phenomenology's founding 'father'
(Laverty, 2003). His was a 'transcendental' phenomenology as he was
interested in the essential experience of things and human consciousness.
Husserl developed phenomenology as the rigorous, "scientific study of
things as they appear to be" (Pernecky & Jamal, 2010, p. 1063), so his
approach aligns with the positivist paradigm. In contrast, Heidegger is
credited with the philosophical turn to an 'existential' phenomenology with
his interest in "understanding humans as existential beings" (Pernecky &
Jamal, p. 1064). Heideggerian phenomenology is a way of uncovering and
interpreting people's situated experiences in the world, thus it fits within the
interpretive paradigm.

Research paradigm	*Philosopher*
Positivist	Edmund Husserl
Post-positivist	Maurice Merleau-Ponty
Interpretivist	Martin Heidegger
Constructivist	Alfred Schütz
Deconstructivist	Jacques Derrida

This chapter is formed around a Heideggerian mode of doing interpretive phenomenology. As the chapter progresses, you will recognize how understanding the
philosophy guides the research question, methodology, and methods. Interpretive
phenomenology sits within the philosophical horizon of hermeneutics, the interpretation of text (Gadamer, 1975/2004), as a way of thinking about understanding
phenomena. Its roots reach back to ancient Greece to a well-known philosopher,
Socrates. In brief, Socrates engaged in conversations with his disciples by assuming a naïve stance on a topic and asking simple questions. Gaps in knowledge
were uncovered and understanding was clarified through questioning and questioning further (Gadamer, 1975/2004). You will recognize this mode of exploring notions when data gathering is discussed later in the chapter. In bringing the
interpretive tradition to studying human engagement (Dreyfus, 1991), Heidegger
was influenced by Dilthey, an earlier German philosopher who moved hermeneutics beyond interpreting written texts to interpreting human thought and lived
experience (Thorne & Collocott, 1974). So let us get closer to what is important
by moving on from interpretive phenomenology as a philosophy to thinking about
it as guiding research methodology.

As a field of inquiry, interpretive phenomenology is the study of how "something
appears or manifests itself" (King, 2001, p. 109). In other words, it studies phenomena as they exist in the world. In colloquial terms, a phenomenon is any observable

fact or occurrence of something. From a Heideggerian perspective, however, a phenomenon is something which is not self-evident; it is taken-for-granted or concealed in some way. It may appear or show itself, hinting at what the phenomenon is, but what it 'is' remains hidden. It is only because the thing itself is concealed that a phenomenological approach is needed (Inwood, 1999). Therefore, doing phenomenology calls for the researcher's thoughtful effort in order to go beyond his or her already held 'knowledge' of things, as these tend to get in the way of understanding what 'is' (Diekelmann, 2005). In my study, I assumed the ubiquitous nature of aging meant the phenomenon of being aged in the everyday was taken-for-granted and therefore 'hidden' from view. Interpretive phenomenology is, therefore, about bringing a thing that is ordinarily hidden into the light. Or as Heidegger (1927/1962) defined it, it is a way of letting "that which shows itself be seen from itself" (p. 58). While this may sound obscure, it simply means that doing phenomenology is about getting as close as possible to understanding what the thing 'is', its meaning, and not simply how it appears or what it seems to be. It illuminates the enduring nature of something. Hence, doing interpretive phenomenology is an ontological mode of inquiry in which the researcher lets something of the phenomenon be seen through language (Gadamer, 1975/2004), through participants' stories of lived experiences. For example, by inviting participants' stories about doing everyday activities following a stroke, researchers have thrown some light on the phenomenon of apraxia (Arntzen & Elstad, 2013).

Ontology

Rather than interpretive phenomenology seeking to understand how people come to know things in the world (epistemology), it seeks to interpret and thus understand the being, or ontology, of everyday human existence (Inwood, 1999). It is a questioning about what it is that fundamentally makes the hidden phenomenon 'what it is'; or in Heidegger's (1927/1962) words, "its Being-what-it-is" (p. 67) and how it appears in the context of everyday life. In my study, I sought to understand the 'being' of being aged. In the midst of burgeoning empirical knowledge about age and aging, I assumed that ontological understanding was usually overlooked.

Defining the topic

Knowing what draws one to the topic of interest is a task for the phenomenological researcher and is important as it aligns with the interpretive phenomenological assumption that the inquirer's pre-understandings cannot be 'bracketed' and put to one side (Heidegger, 1927/1962). Having someone interview the researcher about his or her 'pre-understandings' on the topic of interest is a good way to start, prior to fully reviewing the literature and gathering any data. When I was interviewed by my research supervisor, I talked about my family history, experiences with my grandparents, and of being an occupational therapist. I reflected on what I 'already knew' about aging and being aged from watching, working with, and talking to elders in my community. Textbox 5.2 is an extract from my 1-hour 'pre-understandings interview'.

Textbox 5.2   Example from a pre-understandings interview

When asked about what drew me to my study, I remembered spending time with eight older New Zealanders as they went about doing what they liked to do in a day. Billie took me with her to the zoo on her day as a volunteer Zoo Host. She said the meaning for her was in knowing and sharing knowledge about the many reptiles, birds, and other species. And I joined John in his garage workshop as he hand-crafted a croquet mallet. For him, the meaning was in handling and sculpting the recycled native timbers as well as solving construction problems. The 8 vignettes I gathered became the center-piece of a theoretical conference presentation on aging and the meaning of everyday occupations which enliven the human spirit. By all accounts, the presentation was successful. Yet I was left with a lingering question: Were the stories about enjoyable occupations so compelling that I neglected something as commonplace as how they experienced being the age they were in the context of everyday occupational engagement? In each encounter, I had simply accepted their being aged and looked elsewhere for meaning.

Through transcribing and reflecting on my stories I came to understand more than why I was drawn to the topic; it allowed me to hear the lens I might intuitively bring to questioning participants and interpreting the data. As the study progressed, it enabled me to see when I needed to step back, open up new questions, and let new understandings show. Reflecting on how pre-understandings are influencing thinking, then taking account of them as best as possible when gathering and analyzing data is part of methodological trustworthiness.

The literature review for a phenomenological study might be done in two phases: an initial search to scope the field and identify the knowledge gap/s, with a major search being done once a study's findings are analyzed. Such an approach allows topic definition early in the process and helps the researcher to later stay open to meanings emerging from the data itself. While a classic method might be followed for the main literature review, and is adequate for honors dissertations or Masters' theses, philosophical integrity guides the phenomenologist to uncover the meanings that already exist in the literature regarding the phenomenon of interest. Sources of existing meaning can include scientific literature as well as novels, journals, and poetry. My main literature review, after data analysis, revealed 'being aged' as already meaning a biological phenomenon (Markson, 2003); an outward appearance such as graying hair (Calasanti, 2005), a social category (Degnen, 2007), being wise (Randall & Kenyon, 2004), being decrepit or frail (Johannesen, Petersen, & Avlund, 2004), as well as being a lived experience. The latter were evidenced in a few first-hand accounts of aging (Busch, 1991; Maclean, 2000) and in phenomenological research (Heikkinen, 2004; Nilsson, Sarvimaki, & Ekman, 2000). I noticed that participant quotes in the research publications mostly contained generalized stories about aging rather than particular stories of events 'as they were lived'. These general stories showed how research participants thought about being aged, rather than experiences themselves. I elaborate on this point later in the chapter.

Asking phenomenological questions

The research question defines the identified gap in knowledge, the thing worth understanding, and should name the phenomenon of interest. For my study, it was 'being aged' in the context of everyday life. The question itself will be recognizable as opening an interpretive phenomenological inquiry.

Interpretive phenomenology is a suitable mode of inquiry when little is known about the 'hidden' phenomenon of interest. Phenomenological questions are often 'what' questions; exploring what the experience of something is, such as, what is the lived experience of occupational gaps when doing everyday occupations in the first year following a stroke? (Eriksson & Tham, 2010). Or they may be 'what' questions in relation to what the phenomenon means to those who experience it, such as, what is "the meaning of religion and/or spirituality for people living with a diagnosis of schizophrenia?" (Smith & Suto, 2012, p. 77). Phenomenological questions might also be 'how' questions (Smythe, 2011), yet always in relation to exploring how the phenomenon of interest appears or announces itself in the midst of lived experiences; such as exploring "how do elders experience being aged in their everyday lives?" (Wright-St Clair, 2012, p. 1). A 'why' question has no place in interpretive phenomenology (Smythe, 2011). Once the question is defined, the quest is to determine who to gather 'lived experience' stories from.

Recruitment and sampling

Recruitment for a phenomenological study is almost always purposive as the researcher seeks to identify potential participants with experiences of the phenomenon of interest. How much experience is enough is a considered guess. For example, Arntzen and Elstad (2013) decided at least 1 week post-stroke reasonable for participants' everyday 'experiences' of apraxia. Conversely, Smith and Suto (2012) decided 6 months of 'living with schizophrenia', including at least two hospital admissions, was adequate experience. I set my 'experience of being aged' criterion at 70 years and over for Māori and 80 for non-Māori, respecting the average longevity discrepancy (Crothers, 2003). In reality, it may be informative to recruit some people who have enough and some who have a lot of experience of the thing of interest. The purpose of participant diversity is for deepening thinking about the phenomenon, never for comparative analysis (Smythe, 2011). Methods for locating potential participants will vary, yet will always have the same aim – to access those with a rich experience of the phenomenon. Phenomenology suits direct recruitment, such as advertising in frequented locations or indirect, like inviting community workers or health practitioners to pass on information about the study. Snowball sampling may be appropriate once recruitment has started, particularly when participants are hard to locate. I reasoned that the living context might matter, so only sought participants living in private residences. As a non-Māori researcher, I used two different methods. Non-Māori were recruited using the general electoral roll enabling purposively selection by age, gender, and type of residence. I then sent participant information and a consent form directly to each person. In recruiting Māori, I partnered with a local Māori community health and social service. The service's employed Kaumatua (respected elder) identified those eligible and visited them to talk about the study and gain their consent if interested. Only then did he introduce me.

But doing phenomenology is not a matter of going out, recruiting all participants, gathering all the data, and then analyzing it. To allow thinking along the way, a rolling recruitment method can be implemented. It is best to recruit only one, or a few participants, at a time so each participant's data can be interpreted before interviewing the next participant. Ideally, recruitment continues until it feels like no new notions are emerging, allowing deep interpretation of what the phenomenon means. Up to eight participants will likely be adequate for master's degree students, or up to 20 for doctoral students (Smythe, 2011). Working full-time on my study, I sent recruitment information to a few potential participants at a time and conducted about one interview a month, giving me time to collect, transcribe, and interpret each person's data. In the end, I recruited four Māori aged 71 to 93 and 11 non-Māori aged 80 to 97. Fifteen participants yielded plenty of rich data, but not so much that I became overwhelmed.

Data collection methods

Individual interview is likely to be the data gathering method of choice because "the aim of phenomenology is to transform lived experience into a textual expression" (van Manen, 2001, p. 36). It is within the one-on-one guided conversation (van Manen, 2001) that space is opened up to deeply exploring participants' experiences through stories. It is congruent with the philosophical way of questioning and questioning further and should feel more like an engaging discussion (Johnson, 2002; Warren, 2002) than a question-and-answer interview. Taking a semistructured approach, using a guideline of topics and/or questions, will allow for new questions and notions to emerge within and across the interviews.

Philosophically, it is assumed the ontology, or being, of a hidden human phenomenon can "manifest itself in experience" (Gadamer, 1975/2004, p. 57); hence, the inquiry aims to elicit the telling of experiential stories 'as they were lived'. The researcher aims to evoke prereflective or primordial stories, of particular moments or events (Harman, 2007) rather than generalized or interpretive comments (Bergum, 1991; van Manen, 2001), as illustrated in Textbox 5.3. It is the storied, or textual, accounts of in-the-moment experiences that hold the potential to throw new light on the hidden phenomenon. Collectively, they let an understanding of the whole meaning build (Gadamer, 1975/2004). Asking open questions allows possibilities for participants to say things that could not be anticipated by the researcher. In my study, I invited each participant to "tell me about yesterday". What was said usually hinted at many potential stories about being aged in the everyday. I encouraged stories to continue by asking "then what happened?" And, I invited particular occupational stories; for example, "tell me about the last time you were out in the garden". When it suited, I invited the person to "tell me about being [his/her chronological age]" which always opened up new conversational pathways to follow. To elicit going beyond a story's surface, I would use the person's words, such as "say more about being 'too busy to get old'. "

Textbox 5.3   Example of phenomenological questioning

At age 91 Tom is his wife's main carer; Rosie has dementia.

Tom: *Well, we have been everywhere and done everything, and yet we can't get about like we used to. I don't really get out at all now. We can only go out in the car but we can't go far.*

Tell me about the last time you went out?

Tom: *We went out yesterday. It's just about having a break. It's more or less to take Rosie out and have an ice cream, because Rosie likes her ice cream. I bought the jelly tip ice creams on the way. I took a couple of wee plastic bowls and a tea towel; I spread them out in the car. Then I broke the ice creams up and put them in the wee bowls because they are a bit messy to eat otherwise and Rosie takes a bit longer. We just sat in the car.*

Beyond gathering stories of particular moments and events, interpretive phenomenology gives scope for eliciting participants' interpretation of things (refer to Textbox 5.4). I invited participants' thoughts on things by asking questions like, "What makes a good day for you now?" and "How would you define being aged?" In the flow of the research interview, participant stories are often a blend of prereflective, lived experiences and interpretations of why things are as they are.

Textbox 5.4   Example of interpretive questioning

Mary had already said she didn't 'like getting old' in her story about being "very, very fit" until age 83.

You said earlier you don't like getting old.

Mary: *Yes sometimes I feel a bit old. Oh quite a few times I have felt a bit old. I don't remember any special times, but I would like to be as fit as I was.*

What about times when you think you are not so old?

Mary: *I realise I am very lucky to be as well as I am at 91. I have one hour a week of home help to do the vacuuming and things like that because I am fit enough when I am upright but it is the half bent position when my back bothers me. I don't do the gardening or the vacuuming because I can't be half bent.*

Keeping a reflective journal is congruent with the methodology. It is a way of recording events and observations, as well as emerging thoughts. I wrote down the things I noticed soon after each interview (Textbox 5.5). My reflexive accounts of the person's everyday, his or her occupations and histories became the contextual ground for the research text itself. I also reflected on my 'being a phenomenological researcher' as a way of building competence.

Textbox 5.5   Example of reflective journaling

After my second interview with a Māori participant I wrote:

> The Kaumatua invites me to meet Ella first over a cup of tea. He is outside her house when I arrive and he leads me through the carport to the rear entry. The ranch slider is open and Ella comes to the door. She is very welcoming and insists I shouldn't take off my shoes as we enter into the lounge. I offer my small gift of food. Ella is 93 and I am struck by how petite she is and her gray-stockinged legs look almost fragile between her black slippers and knitted black skirt. Her jumper is black with bold multiple textures and patterns. Ella's collar-length hair is dark gray and thinning and she has it loose. . . .

Data analysis methods

Interpretive phenomenological analysis is an inductive, iterative process. There is no one-way of doing the interpretation, but certain features should be evident in the methods. Importantly, analysis begins with and continues alongside data collection; one informs the other. This is because the thinking about what the text is saying and the thinking about what it means begins the moment data gathering begins. It is grounded in the data. Ongoing analysis will reveal new ways of thinking about the phenomenon of interest and new questions to ask.

I think of transcribing the data as part of the analysis. Listening, and re-listening, to the stories while typing up the transcripts is a way of dwelling with the interview data and of beginning to engage fully with it. It assists a deep familiarity with the text. As I transcribed I often heard things I had not noticed during the conversation itself, informing questions for subsequent interviews. The analysis progresses with drawing out stories, or anecdotes, from the data that say something about experiencing the phenomenon of interest. I prefer to talk about 'anecdotes', implying a particular type of story (van Manen, 2001) compared to 'stories' which can suggest a fictional account of something (Caelli, 2001).

Drawing out the anecdotes

The interpretive phenomenological researcher's task is to draw out the lived experience anecdotes from the interview transcripts. In their telling of the private life, coherent anecdotes hold the potential to show that which is ordinarily hidden in the everyday. They can make "comprehensible some notion that easily eludes us" (van Manen, 2001, p. 116). So, it works best to return the anecdotes to participants for verification. Because interview transcripts are an accurate record of what was said they show the disarray of conversations because "nobody talks in prose" (Richardson, 2002, p. 879). One story might start then lead off into another, before being revisited somewhere in the flow of dialog. Sentences may be incomplete or grammatically incorrect making them clumsy to read; thus, the messiness of transcribed conversational text can act to conceal its meaning (Caelli, 2001). I drew out the anecdotes by pulling the pieces together when a story was disjointed. When repetitions in the text did not add to the meaning, such as showing emphasis, I removed duplications, and tidied grammatical structures so that the meaning was not lost in awkward language, leaving the meanings untouched. Textbox 5.6 contains one coherent anecdote drawn from my text. Data unrelated to the phenomenon of interest can simply be left behind in the transcripts. I compiled each participant's collected anecdotes into a booklet and returned them for verification.

Beyond the methodological rigor this method offers, there were unexpected benefits. One participant, who had said he was ready for his time in this world to come to an end passed his collection on to his daughter. He told me she read it a few times and she cried. Then he passed it on to his doctor to read because his doctor was not listening to his voiced readiness to go. Another passed his collection around his numerous children and grandchildren so they might understand how his everyday was.

Textbox 5.6   Drawing out an anecdote

This anecdote was drawn from a long section of text when I asked Ella 'do you remember a moment recently when time seemed to go by slowly?' It reveals some in-the-moment experiences as well as some interpretations of what is going on:

Since I came out of hospital Rosemarie has been teaching the children at dance class and she had about 40 yards of pink denim given to her which she used for all the costumes. She made the six girls' skirts, each with different black lace, and I ironed them all. See, if anything is going on like that, all of a sudden something happens and I have got something to do. I will just show you the skirts. I won't pull them all out. They looked beautiful. I ironed them. You see these things come up, whereas if I was in a home or even with my other daughter, this would never come up. What would I do? With Rosemarie, she has an idea and I can do it. So these things come up; it is something different. Well, each day I can do more. It is not that I am longing to do things, but I don't want to be sitting and doing nothing and thinking about nothing. [Ella, 93]

There is no 'ideal' number of anecdotes to draw from a transcript. It is up to the researcher to work diligently through the text. It is time to move on to analyzing the data once there is a sense of knowing all anecdotes saying something about the phenomenon of interest are captured. It took me about a month as a full-time student to work with each participant's anecdotes.

Interpreting the anecdotes

Again, there is no one right way of doing the analyzing but it has one essential feature; it is interpretive. It is a thinking engagement (Harman, 2007; Smythe, Ironside, Sims, Swenson, & Spence, 2008). Interpretive phenomenological analysis is not a thematic analysis of the content (Smythe, 2011); it is a way of thinking about the meanings within the text. In the play of thinking, the gaze is always directed toward the phenomenon of interest. van Manen's (2001) 'selective reading' approach guides a way of listening to or reading an anecdote several times and asking "what statement(s) or phrase(s) seem particularly essential or revealing about the phenomenon or experience being described?" (p. 93). This text is then highlighted in some way. This is when thinking through writing comes into its own. Rather than pondering the meaning and then writing it down, it is more fruitful to just start writing about an anecdote and its text that seems particularly revealing. Writing begets thinking. And, it is within the thinking that the 'interpretive leap' (Smythe, 2011) happens; when suddenly something otherwise concealed shows itself in some way. Being true to the methodology means the researcher's interpretations are the researcher's (Gadamer, 1975/2004), as it is the researcher who hears many stories and who brings his or her own history and pre-understandings into the interpretive play. The interpretations cannot move away from the text itself, but they do go beyond the text's content. Philosophical writings can be drawn on to deepen interpretations. Interpretive writings are not returned to the participants but a summary of the findings may be.

When I engaged in data analysis, I attempted to approach the anecdotal text with a sense of wonderment at, and a not-knowing about, what lay before me. My experience was of being receptive and attentive to the text by dwelling with it in an uninterrupted way (Gadamer, 1975/2004), going backward and forward between the whole anecdote and the highlighted phrases. The writing opened up listening beyond the words (Diekelmann, 2001) allowing possible meanings to emerge. Textbox 5.7 illustrates a way of interpretive writing.

Textbox 5.7   Interpreting the text

I wrote several pages when first interpreting Ella's anecdote about ironing the six denim skirts. What follows is an extract, showing my use of the highlighted (italicized) text and my interpretive leaps in understanding:

In the midst of talking, Ella notices how being with Rosemarie means *all of a sudden something happens* in her day. Unexpectedly, something presents itself and she has *got something to do*. Rosemarie invites her mother's involvement. The situation holds an expectancy which lets Ella become involved. Being there means Ella is opened up to possibilities in her day. The 'there' is not the place itself, in a spatial sense, but "the space it opens up and illuminates" (Inwood, 1999, p. 42). In other words, the context itself is revealing, lighting up possibilities for engaging. On this occasion, Ella's 'thereness' meant the ironing, which was not there before, *came up* for her. The new possibilities come as a surprise as if "the environment announces itself afresh" (Heidegger, 1927/1962, p. 105).

Interpreting and further data gathering continues until the whole research text is assembled. It is then time to analyze across the texts, to interpret what experiencing the phenomenon of interest means. Making drawings or capturing ideas in poetry about what stands out throughout the interpretive process can be helpful ways of trying to see and capture what matters.

Interpreting the meaning

This phase of the research journey is one of moving from being in an interpretive engagement with the subjective anecdotes to a broader reflection on the phenomenon itself. It is a mode of thinking across the whole research text and of writing a "phenomenological textual description" (van Manen, 2001, p. 106) that moves toward interpreting meaning. It is a mode of wondering about what is brought into the light and what remains in darkness. Hermeneutically, it is a continual movement from considering the whole research text to taking account of its parts, ensuring that one is reflected in the other. Particular anecdotes that show as rich illustrations of each notion are drawn in (Diekelmann, 2001) and together say something of the meaning. This is where van Manen's (2001) 'wholistic reading approach' may be useful; drawing out the particular anecdotes and interpretive writings from the whole research text that "capture the fundamental meaning or main significance of the text as a whole" (p. 93). In my study, I aimed to unveil the harmony between the textual parts and the interpretive whole. What showed through was that the meaning of being aged is its ordinariness within the everyday, clustering around four main notions: Being in the everyday, being with others, experiencing the unaccustomed, and aging just is (Wright-St Clair, 2008).

Rigor and ethics

Annells' (1999) four criteria for evaluating phenomenological research is a useful framework for determining trustworthiness. First, evaluating whether the study is 'understandable and appreciable'. Clear, simple language that fits with the methodology should be used, and the interpreted meanings made clear. Second, whether 'an understandable inquiry process' is evident? A 'trail' of philosophically sound methodological decisions should be evident in the research process described. Third, the 'usefulness' of the outcome is judged. Even though interpretive phenomenology is not applied research, it should lead to potentially useful practice implications. And fourth, evaluating the 'appropriateness' of the inquiry. In essence, it is judging the "congruency of the approach to the research question" (Annells, 1999, p. 11) that it names the phenomenological approach used, it explores lived experiences of a named phenomenon and it interprets the experiential meaning.

Critiquing phenomenological studies

Incongruences in 'phenomenological' studies often show in the nature of the interview questions, participant quotes reporting generalized experiences and 'perceptions' of the phenomenon, including data that lose their gaze on the phenomenon of interest, and thematic coding of narrative content. It may be a reflection of poor writing up, or, more likely, it suggests the researcher's need to better understand the philosophical underpinnings of interpretive phenomenology. Hence, it is important to ask some critical questions (Textbox 5.8) when reading phenomenological studies.

Textbox 5.8   Critiquing phenomenological studies – things to look for

1   Is the *ontological* nature of the methodology clearly stated and justified?
2   Do the authors state what *variant of phenomenology* is being used?
3   Is the *phenomenon of interest* clearly stated?
4   Is the research question aimed at exploring *lived experience* or *meaning* of the phenomenon?
5   Is adequate *experience of the phenomenon* evident in the participant inclusion criteria?
6   Is it evident stories about *particular experiential moments* were gathered?
7   Are participants' *interpretations* of things also evident?
8   Have the authors described how they *analyzed each participant's stories*?
9   Have philosophical writings been used to deepen interpretations?
10   Have the authors described how they *analyzed across the whole text*?
11   Have the authors used *reflective journaling* as part of rigor?
12   Is the *meaning* of the phenomenon of interest interpreted and described?

Application to occupational science

Occupational science shares a philosophical harmony with interpretive phenomenology (Reed, Hocking, & Smythe, 2011; Wilding & Whiteford, 2005). Given occupational science's aim of understanding the occupational essence of 'being' human (Wilcock, 2006), the ontological nature of interpretive phenomenology in understanding the 'being' of things lines up effortlessly. Phenomenology is under-pinned by the idea that existing in a context "with particular things and estab-lished ways of doing things" (Wrathall, 2005, p. 15), rather than thinking ability, is what makes humans human. As an interpretive phenomenologist, Heidegger's "thinking dwelled in the complex realm of ordinary, everyday human existence" (Wright-St Clair & Smythe, 2012, p. 36). Therefore, the ontology, or 'being', of being engaged in doing is the rich turf in which human occupation is grounded. The next philosophical alignment seems equally as compelling. That is, mounting empirical knowledge about the forms, functions, and meanings of people's every-day occupations is a primary focus of studying human occupation from an occu-pational science standpoint (Zemke & Clark, 1996). In congruence, interpreting a phenomenon's meaning is the purpose of interpretive phenomenology. Lastly, if occupational science's endeavor is to build knowledge of both the 'observ-able' and the 'phenomenological' dimensions (Clark & Lawlor, 2009) of human occupation, then interpretive phenomenology's harmony is evident through its exploration of being occupied as it is experienced by people, individually and collectively in the world. Accepting "there is not one but many truths, or multiple realities about occupations and the occupational nature of humans, this opens the way for studying the phenomenological aspects" (Wright-St Clair & Hocking, 2013, p. 83) of being occupied.

My study's interpretive findings contribute to the occupational science world through illuminating something of what being aged means when going about the everyday in advanced age. Occupationally, four things showed as mattering (Wright-St Clair, Kerse, & Smythe, 2011). Ordinariness matters. Having things seem 'as they usually are' in advanced age is about carrying on; getting on with, being absorbed in, and doing things which are there to be done. It keeps things in their place and holds things together. Purposefulness matters. Having a purpose is a reason for being; it gives meaning. It shows in doing things for the sake of others, in passing something on, and being ready for leaving something behind. Memories matter. In being aged, memories offer a 'nearness' to people, places, things done, and times gone by, even when alone. The dwelling place matters, as this is where everyday life is encountered. Being in everyday places which invoke being involved matters (Wright-St Clair, 2012); it is about having occupations that draw one into the day; occupations that reflect back who one was, is, and will be in advanced age.

Application to occupational therapy

Phenomenological research findings alone will not evidence what clinically effec-tive occupational therapy practice should look like, but they will evidence what matters to people as they go about their occupationally contextualized lives. Lived experience data "can reveal deeper interpretations of people's engagement in eve-ryday occupations" (Wright-St Clair & Smythe, 2012, p. 26) and get closer to understanding the meaning of things for them. In accord, interpretive phenomenology can inform how occupational therapists think about engaging in dialog with the people they work with. Engaging is a way of inviting stories about being in life's ordinary and unfamiliar moments and events as lived, of openly questioning, and questioning further to elicit new understandings (Wright-St Clair et al., 2011). It is a way of fully " 'listening' for that which is hidden from the outside… [implying that] practitioners who listen in different ways, beyond the self-evident and the taken-for-granted, will have richer understandings to call on when making inferences and decisions" (Wright-St Clair & Smythe, 2012, p. 35). And, it is knowing that each practice encounter, despite being with the same person/s, is unique to doing this occupation, in this context at this time (Harman, 2007). While such a way of practice will reap its own benefits for the recipients of occupational therapy, and occupational therapists themselves, being clinically effective matters. To this end, phenomenological data may be used to complement, or deepen, quantitative empirical research data within a mixed methods study, offering the potential for stronger evidence-based practice results. Findings from a study of adults with spinal cord injury lived experience stories of going about their day informed subsequent, and on-going, projects aimed at developing theory on how pressure ulcers develop, to then test cost-effective, occupation-focused interventions in clinical trials (Clark et al., 2006). As with all researches, a robustly designed and implemented phenomenological study holds the greatest potential for yielding fruitful results.

Personal reflections

Heidegger (1927/1962) said "to think is to confine yourself to a single thought that one day stands still like a star in the world's sky" (p. 4). Where I found my place in being an interpretive phenomenologist was in discovering a point of relative stillness in thinking amid the tossing and turning movements toward understanding my data. I was always wondering 'what is the meaning of being aged' amidst everyday life in advanced age. Dwelling was stepping close and listening in to anecdotes and evocative phrases, dwelling was stepping back to see things in their wholeness. It was a distilling of the meaning of being aged in the everyday from all that was said and not said. Entering into the space of a participant's usual world was like discovering a treasure trove.

> The things ordinary to each person and each space appeared to me uniquely extraordinary and called forth my wondering. Each thing, each moment, told its own story; approaching down the pathway darkened by overhanging creepers, gazing upon the wheelbarrow storing firewood in the lounge, noticing the piano taking up much of the room, looking into the tiny black and white photographs. And there was an unspoken wonderfulness which radiated from within each person; it showed in the eyes, the smile, the hands. It was extraordinary how much I was drawn to 'hear'. (Wright-St Clair, 2008, pp. 202–203)

For me, learning to be a phenomenologist was a privileged place to dwell.

Summary

The doing of interpretive phenomenology is as much to do with becoming a phenomenologist as it is with the doing phenomenology. It means reading philosophy, in this case some of the works of Martin Heidegger, Hans-Georg Gadamer, and others who interpreted their works. It means 'knowing' what the phenomenon of interest is and gathering storied data on people's lived experiences to come closer to understanding what it means. It means being at peace with the slowness of thinking and writing, and re-thinking and re-writing and understanding emerges. It means being comfortable with uncertainty and the tentativeness of knowledge. This chapter has mapped one rigorous way of doing interpretive phenomenology, illustrated by examples from one New Zealand study. While there is no one right way, it is beholden upon the researcher to show in his or her writing how the particular philosophical underpinnings guided the research methods. Interpretive phenomenology offers a way of doing research that aligns with occupational science's fundamental tenets. For the occupational therapist, it informs a way of being in practice and of building sound evidence for practice.

References

Annells, M. (1999). Evaluating phenomenology: Usefulness, quality and philosophical foundations. *Nurse Researcher, 6*(3), 5–19.

Arntzen, C., & Elstad, I. (2013). The bodily experience of apraxia in everyday activities: A phenomenological study. *Disability and Rehabilitation, 35*(1), 63–72. doi:10.3109/0 9638288.2012.687032.

Bergum, V. (1991). Being a phenomenological researcher. In J. Morse (Ed.), *Qualitative nursing research* (pp. 55–71). Newbury Park, CA: Sage.

Busch, G. (1991). *You are my darling Zita.* Auckland, New Zealand: Godwit Press.

Caelli, K. (2001). Engaging with phenomenology: Is it more of a challenge than it needs to be? *Qualitative Health Research, 11*(2), 273–281.

Calasanti, T. (2005). Ageism, gravity, and gender: Experiences of aging bodies. *Generations, 29*(3), 8–12.

Clark, F., Jackson, J., Scott, M., Atkins, M., Uhles-Tanaka, M., & Rubayi, S. (2006). Data-based models of how pressure ulcers develop in daily-living contexts of adults with spinal cord injury. *Archives of Physical Medicine and Rehabilitation, 87*(11), 1516–1525. doi:10.1016/j.apmr.2006.08.329.

Clark, F., & Lawlor, M. (2009). The making and mattering of occupational science. In E. B. Crepeau, E. S. Cohn, & B. A. Schell (Eds.), *Willard & Spackman's occupational therapy* (11th ed., pp. 2–14). Philadelphia, PA: Lippincott Williams & Wilkins.

Crothers, C. (2003). Maori well-being and disparity in Tamaki-Makaurau. *New Zealand Population Review, 29*(1), 111–129.

Degnen, C. (2007). Minding the gap: The construction of old age and oldness amongst peers. *Journal of Aging Studies, 21*(1), 69–80.

Diekelmann, J. (2005). The retrieval of method: The method of retrieval. In N. Diekelmann (Series Ed.) & P. M. Ironside (Vol. Ed.), *Beyond method: Philosophical conversations in health care research and scholarship* (Vol. IV, pp. 3–57). Madison, WI: The University of Wisconsin Press.

Diekelmann, N. (2001). Narrative pedagogy: Heideggerian hermeneutical analyses of lived experiences of students, teachers, and clinicians (teaching and learning). *Advances in Nursing Science, 23*(3), 53–71.

Dreyfus, H. L. (1991). *Being-in-the-world: A commentary on Heidegger's being and time, division I.* Cambridge, MA: The MIT Press.

Eriksson, G., & Tham, T. (2010). The meaning of occupational gaps in everyday life in the first year after stroke. *OTJR: Occupation, Participation and Health, 30*(4), 184–192. doi:10.3928/15394492–20091123–01.

Gadamer, H.-G. (1975/2004). *Truth and method* (J. Weinsheimer & D. G. Marshall, Trans., 2nd, Rev ed.). London, UK: Continuum.

Harman, G. (2007). *Heidegger explained: From phenomenon to thing.* Chicago: Open Court.

Heidegger, M. (1927/1962). *Being and time* (J. Macquarrie & E. Robinson, Trans., 7th ed.). Oxford, UK: Blackwell Publishers.

Heikkinen, R. L. (2004). The experience of ageing and advanced old age: A ten-year follow-up. *Ageing and Society, 24*(4), 567–582. doi:10.1017/S0144686X04001837.

Inwood, M. (1999). *A Heidegger dictionary.* Malden, MA: Blackwell Publishing.

Johannesen, A., Petersen, J., & Avlund, K. (2004). Satisfaction in everyday life for frail 85-year-old adults: A Danish population study. *Scandinavian Journal of Occupational Therapy, 11*(1), 3–11. doi:10.1080/11038120410019045.

Johnson, J. M. (2002). In-depth interviewing. In J. F. Gubrium & J. A. Holstein (Eds.), *Handbook of interview research: Context & method* (pp. 103–119). Thousand Oaks, CA: Sage.

King, M. (2001). *A guide to Heidegger's being and time.* Albany, NY: State University of New York Press.

Laverty, S. M. (2003). Hermeneutic phenomenology and phenomenology: A comparison of historical and methodological considerations. *International Journal of Qualitative Methods, 2*(3), 21–35.

Maclean, J. (Ed.). (2000). *At the end of the day: Ten New Zealanders in their 80s reflect on life in old age.* Wellington, New Zealand: Steele Roberts Ltd.

Markson, E. W. (2003). *Social gerontology today: An introduction.* Los Angeles, CA: Roxbury Publishing Company.

Nilsson, M., Sarvimaki, A., & Ekman, S.-L. (2000). Feeling old: Being in a phase of transition in later life. *Nursing Inquiry, 7*(1), 41–49.

Pernecky, T., & Jamal, T. (2010). (Hermeneutic) Phenomenology in tourism studies. *Annals of Tourism Research, 37*(4), 1055–1075. doi:10.1016/j.annals.2010.04.002.

Randall, W. L., & Kenyon, G. M. (2004). Time, story, and wisdom: Emerging themes in narrative gerontology. *Canadian Journal on Aging, 23*(4), 333–346.

Reed, K. D., Hocking, C. S., & Smythe, L. A. (2011). Exploring the meaning of occpation: The case for phenomenology. *Canadian Journal of Occupational Therapy, 78*, 303–310. doi:10.2182/cjot.2011.78.5.5.

Richardson, L. (2002). Poetic representation of interviews. In J. F. Gubrium & J. A. Holstein (Eds.), *Handbook of interview research: Context & method* (pp. 877–891). Thousand Oaks, CA: Sage.

Smith, S., & Suto, M. J. (2012). Religious and/or spiritual practices: Extending spiritual freedom to people with schizophrenia. *Canadian Journal of Occupational Therapy, 79*(2), 77–85. doi:10.2182/cjot.2012.79.2.3.

Smythe, E. A. (2011). From beginning to end: How to do hermeneutic interpretive phenomenology. In G. Thomson, F. Dykes, & S. Downe (Eds.), *Qualitative research in midwifery and childbirth* (pp. 35–54). London, UK/New York, NY: Routledge.

Smythe, E. A., Ironside, P. M., Sims, S. L., Swenson, M. M., & Spence, D. G. (2008). Doing Heideggerian hermeneutic research: A discussion paper. *International Journal of Nursing Studies, 45*, 1389–1397. doi:10.1016/j.ijnurstu.2007.09.005.

Thorne, J. O., & Collocott, T. C. (Eds.). (1974). *Chambers biographical dictionary* (Rev ed.). Edinburgh, Scotland: W & R Chambers Ltd.

van Manen, M. (2001). *Researching lived experience: Human science for an action sensitive pedagogy* (2nd ed.). London, UK/Ontario, Canada: The Althouse Press.

Warren, C. A. B. (2002). Qualitative interviewing. In J. F. Gubrium & J. A. Holstein (Eds.), *Handbook of interview research: Context & method* (pp. 83–101). Thousand Oaks, CA: Sage.

Wilcock, A. (2006). *An occupational perspective of health* (2nd ed.). Thorofare, NJ: Slack.

Wilding, C., & Whiteford, G. (2005). Phenomenological research: An exploration of conceptual, theoretical, and practical issues. *OTJR: Occupation, Participation and Health, 25*(3), 98–104.

Wrathall, M. (2005). *How to read Heidegger*. London, UK: Granta Books.

Wright-St Clair, V. A. (2008). *'Being aged' in the everyday: Uncovering the meaning through elders' stories* (Doctoral). University of Auckland, Auckland. Retrieved from http://hdl.handle.net/2292/3080. doi:http://hdl.handle.net/2292/3080.

Wright-St Clair, V. A. (2012). Being occupied with what matters in advanced age. *Journal of Occupational Science, 19*(1), 44–53. doi:10.1080/14427591.2011.639135.

Wright-St Clair, V. A., & Hocking, C. (2013). Occupational science: The study of occupation. In B. A. Schell, G. Gillen, & M. Scaffa (Eds.), *Willard & Spackman's occupational therapy* (12th ed., pp. 82–93). Baltimore, MD: Lippincott, Williams & Wilkins.

Wright-St Clair, V. A., Kerse, N., & Smythe, L. (2011). Doing everyday occupations both conceals and reveals the phenomenon of being aged. *Australian Occupational Therapy Journal, 58*(2), 88–94. doi:10.1111/j.1440–1630.2010.00885.x.

Wright-St Clair, V. A., & Smythe, E. A. (2012). Being occupied in the everyday. In M. Cutchin & V. Dickie (Eds.), *Transactional perspectives on occupation* (pp. 25–37). New York, NY: Springer.

Zemke, R., & Clark, F. (1996). *Occupational science: The evolving discipline*. Philadelphia, PA: F.A. Davis.

Further reading

Benner, P. (Ed.). (1994). *Interpretive phenomenology: Embodiment, caring, and ethics in health and illness*. Thousand Oaks, CA: Sage.

Todres, L., & Galvin, K. T. (2012). "In the middle of everywhere": A phenomenological study of mobility and dwelling amongst rural elders. *Phenomenology & Practice, 6*(1), 55–68.

van Manen, M. (Ed.). (2002). *Writing in the dark: Phenomenological studies in interpretive inquiry*. London, UK/Ontario, Canada: Althouse Press.

Websites

http://www.iep.utm.edu/heidegge/
http://www.phenomenologyonline.com/sources/textorium/

6 Narrative methodology

A tool to access unfolding and situated meaning in occupation

Staffan Josephsson and Sissel Alsaker

There has been a growing critique in qualitative methods, over the last decades, regarding the difficulty for traditional qualitative research methods to capture the richness of phenomena in life and how these are lived and experienced (Denzin, 2013; Holstein & Gubrium, 2012). Indeed, qualitative studies tend to portray components and general characteristics of a phenomenon without fully accessing the unfolding and multifaceted character of the presence of phenomena in everyday situations. This evolving discussion has been seen within occupational science and occupational therapy. For example, Frank and Polkinghorne (2010) addressed the development to more nuanced and sensitive qualitative methodologies in occupational therapy while Borell, Nygård, Asaba, Gustavsson, and Hemmingson (2012) reported, based on a review of recent qualitative studies, how most published qualitative studies describe components rather than developing new knowledge on how these components are situated and intersect.

In this chapter, we present narrative methodology and respond to the call for an elaborated and sensitive qualitative inquiry within occupational science and occupational therapy. To present the rich field of a qualitative methodology, such as narrative, in the confines of a chapter is a challenge. There are a multitude of traditions and suggestions on how narrative can be used in qualitative research drawing from diverse theoretical underpinnings. Thus, presenting a short and clear structure for how to use narrative in research, when narrative by itself is about complexity, multitude, and contradictions, is something of an antilogy. In this chapter, our response to the challenge is to ground the methodology we present in specific theory as well as in our current practice, thus giving an example of how narrative theory and methodology can be tailored for use in specific research projects. An example from our own research will be used to demonstrate how narrative methodology can give access to the unfolding, situated, and multifold character of human occupation.

Given that the relation between narrative and action are in the forefront of this chapter, it is logical that resources from Aristotle (1920), Ricoeur (1984a), and Mattingly (1998), central scholars on meaning and action, are the theorists that we draw upon. Further material from a study on narrative in action among women living with chronic rheumatic disease will be our empirical source (Alsaker & Josephsson, 2010).

Background

Narrative is a way to approach and understand meaning in relation to humans and their lives, with the concept of narrative emerging in a variety of ways within different contexts and situations. The term is used in relation to verbal performances at storytelling cafés in the community, as well as when clients talk about their lives in therapeutic practices and, as in this chapter, in discussions on qualitative methodology as a research tool. The use of narrative in these shifting situations and contexts is diverse, and attention needs to be paid to the context within which it is being used. Overall, when the term "narrative" is used, it is first and foremost associated with words, either in the form of verbal storytelling or textual representations, such as in novels or poetry, offering human meaning-making.

In occupational science and occupational therapy, scholars have taken another point of departure, where it is often argued that narrative is not just about words, as used in oral or written language, but is also a useful concept to develop understanding of possible meanings of the actions that make up the everyday lives of humans (Josephsson, Asaba, Jonsson, & Alsaker, 2006). When scholars in occupational science and occupational therapy make such a link between meaning and action they are in good company. Aristotle (1920) made this link in his book on the art of tragedy. He identified human actions as materials that communicate possibilities for humans to create meanings about things encountered in life. For example, when one reads a book or views a theater performance, one reads about or sees people and their actions and the excitement experienced is related to the connections ascribed and causality to what is happening to the actors. As a reader or spectator, one produces images of what is happening in the text or on the stage and tries out different images of how the happenings will develop. In other words, narrative is not only about words it is also about human action. Aristotle and his reasoning on actions were central building blocks when the French philosopher Ricoeur (1984a), more than two thousand years after Aristotle, wrote a series of books linking human meaning-making with action and narrative. Mattingly (1998) is a contemporary scholar contributing to the dialog on narrative, drawing in particular on Ricoeur's writing on narrative in relation to action.

Epistemology

To say that narrative is linked to action is not controversial. To try and tell a story that does not contain any account of action is probably a difficult endeavor. Rather the question is how is narrative linked to action? Maybe it is the action in itself that makes the story become a story? Ricoeur used Aristotle's reasoning on mimesis to build his theory on the links between narrative and action (see Mattingly (1998) and Ricoeur (1991) for a presentation on Aristotle's use of mimesis). Mimesis is a term used by Plato for representation, and Aristotle used the term in a similar way. To put it simply, representation means that something is recognized as similar to something else and can represent that other thing in a more simple or comprehensive way. However, when Ricoeur (1984b) revisited Aristotle's reasoning on mimesis in his work on time and narrative, representation was not the central point. Rather, he argued that the concept of mimesis does not have to portray something as similar to anything; instead, he reasoned that narrative is connected to and embedded within human action. Through the processes of making plots, human beings make links between meaning and action, processes which Ricoeur identified as "emplotment". By making images, people emplot possible links and meanings among available materials, images that contain facts, events, and circumstances that are linked into causal relations and thereby they become possible to understand. In establishing these causal relations possible meanings occur (Alsaker, Bongaardt, & Josephsson, 2009; Josephsson, la Cour, & Jonsson 2007).

Further, in action that is narrative, there is also the presence of suspense or something that is not easy to make a clear sense of. There are several possible plots that can be identified. To understand how this process might work we explore Ricoeur's reasoning further. Action or activity occurs within a context, a context that is recognizable within a particular culture. Such context is located in a particular place that contains objects, materials and often people. Ricoeur identified the mimesis process as being about how people involved in actions understand what is going on within particular places and cultures. How then do people manage to understand or emplot the activity situations in ways that enable them to respond, resonance, and act? According to Ricoeur's mimesis process, people act according to their knowledge of the settings in which they are situated, a knowledge that is based on their experiences of living and acting in specific cultures. Out of this general knowledge, people produce a variety of images regarding the specific acting situation in which they participate. In other words, they emplot their tentative interpretation of what is going on by trying out possible ways of understanding and by imagining possible links and causalities. But these possible stories are not complete – they consist of incidents, occasions, beginnings, and suspense. Given that the situations, environments, and cultures in which people act are complex and dynamic, with multiple enmeshed plots, ongoing action remains evolving, and in suspense with no final emplotment. Different emplotments are at play, and to figure out possibilities within the specific situations people are situated within, they need to act, to continuously play out, and to get responses from the people and circumstances that are meeting them. At this point, the reader might be wondering why all the theory on narrative, action, and meaning is necessary when the chapter is about how to conduct qualitative research guided by a narrative methodology? We contend that when we do narrative analysis we draw on how meaning is enacted and constructed in everyday life. Therefore, we need to ground our methodological choice in theory on meaning-making. There are different traditions on how construction and portrayal of meaning works in practice and researchers need to make a choice on how their study will be grounded within theory. This choice will influence how the subsequent research activities are planned and performed.

Defining the topic

Within guidelines for conducting research, it is often claimed that the first step is to define the problem and based on the problem specify the research question (DePoy & Gitlin, 2011; Holstein & Gubrium, 2012). This is generally very good advice and applicable to narrative methods as well. However, it might be tempting to apply a linear reasoning to the project and, if so, the focus on versatility and complexity would generally be less relevant. Within narrative methodology the process of finding and defining the problem and the specific research question is better viewed as an on-going endeavor throughout the research.

Another central aspect for a narrative study is to know if the methodology is relevant in relation to the problem under investigation. How does one know when narrative methodology is relevant for a study? The question that needs to be asked is whether the study is related to meaning and how meaning is established in everyday situations? The key point here is to ask questions related to "how", rather than to what or why, as the "how" question signals that the generation of knowledge about phenomena that are emerging and relational, rather than descriptions of components and facts. It is the process of how meaning is established and recreated that is to be traced in the narrative analyses. For example, we have been interested in how meaning in everyday occupations is established and revised for women living with chronic health conditions. With this broad area as our starting point, we have refined our focus raising questions such as how four women living with chronic rheumatic conditions related to and communicated moral issues in their everyday occupations (Alsaker & Josephsson, 2011). The issue of morality in relation to meaning and everyday activities stemmed from the research process and will be further illustrated under analysis of data. See Textbox 6.1 for examples of narrative research questions from the published literature.

Textbox 6.1   Examples of narrative research questions

1   What are the dimensions of occupational balance or imbalance for individuals with rheumatoid arthritis? (Stamm et al., 2009)
2   How do women make sense of living with multiple sclerosis? (Wright-St Clair, 2003)
3   How do fathers of children with disabilities represent the experience of engagement in fathering occupations? (Bonsall, 2013)
4   What are older people's experiences of retirement based on active pre-retirement planning? (Hewitt, Howie, & Feldman, 2010)

Generation of data

Generating data in narrative research is not an isolated activity separated from analysis. However, for practical reasons and for ease of access for the reader, we address sampling, data gathering, and analysis of data separately.

Recruitment and sampling

The success of a narrative study depends on accessing rich material. By rich material we mean vivid material offering a multitude of interpretative possibilities, but rich does not mean spectacular nor does it need to be about extreme situations and odd or dramatic events. Rather, data need to be multilayered and evolving. So when identifying participants, it is necessary to find people that are both able and willing to contribute with such significant and rich material. In practice, this often comes down to the time that can be invested in a project as well as the time participants have. More seldom it is about the number of participants. The call for rich material can also serve as a concept sensitizing the researcher when gathering data in a narrative study to ensure that material has quality that is sufficient for a narrative analysis. This reasoning resonates with the anthropological concept of thick descriptions (Geertz, 1973) referring to representations of human behavior that explains not just the behavior, but its context as well, such that the behaviour becomes meaningful to an outsider.

We exemplify this reasoning of sampling with help of our study on women living with chronic conditions. Since the focus of that study was how meaning in everyday activities is established and revised among women living with chronic health conditions, we had chosen to utilize participant observation. This meant that the participants of the study needed to be willing to invite us into their everyday life for a period of time. This was the central criterion for participant inclusion. To get access to participants we recruited through a consumer organization in the local community following the procedures advised by the local ethics committee.

Data collection methods

When narrative is mentioned in relation to qualitative research it is often seen as synonymous to verbal data gathered through interviews. To count as verbal data for a narrative inquiry, data need to be storied, that is, be presented in narrative forms. Storied data need, in line with the theoretical orientation, to be emplotted to reveal possible meanings. One practical way to get storied material when gathering data through interviews is to elicit stories rather than stay with open-ended questions that might lead the interviewee to a focus on descriptive information and facts. One common misunderstanding though is to interpret 'storied' to mean coherent and structured stories with a specific beginning, middle, and end. When telling stories in everyday life, the telling takes an improvisational character with lots of side tracks, pauses, and unfinished lines (Mattingly, 1998). Therefore, the researcher must be skilled and identify potential gaps that arise in the story telling and ask questions that flesh out the details of the story.

When collecting narrative material one needs to decide whether the data collecting context is to be in a one-to-one setting in an office-like environment, in home or work (natural) environments, or whether data will be gathered in fieldwork settings. In the literature, there is abundant argument for collecting narrative material in natural and fieldwork settings, especially when research questions are focused on occupational phenomena (Alsaker et al., 2009) as narratives are about images of how things relate and communicate, and natural surroundings prompt such images. The researcher asks questions which relate to the natural surroundings. For example, when sitting at the kitchen table in the respondent's home, the respondent is more likely to relate incidents and episodes that are connected to how the everyday happens in that home context and will also easily give access to images of earlier experiences in similar settings.

The interview questions need to elicit narrative material in an interview setting. The researcher might start by asking "how" questions relating to how persons live their everyday life. For example, "Please tell me about a few incidents/episodes where you managed your everyday chores well, and the opposite where you had trouble or did not do well". If the answers are very factual ("I make my breakfast cereals alone and eat it by the kitchen table"), the researcher can prompt, "Please tell me more about your morning ritual" or "how do you move from home to work?" often followed by prompts for further reflections such as "Please elaborate on the incidents where you met with your neighbor at the bus stop". When respondents start to talk, a narrative researcher needs to pay close attention to when storied material appears and ask for more elaborations. Narrative material includes emplotments such as "first I did this, and then I thought this, and suddenly I met a friend of mine . . . and she told me that another friend of ours just had . . . . And then you see, we have been friends for a long time . . . . And I was so happy to run into her . . . you have no idea how much fun we had together . . . ".

Observations and particularly participant observations are useful tools for gathering data for narrative analysis if there is a focus on meaning and action. We outlined a theoretical grounding for this statement earlier when arguing that emplotment of possible meaning is not only a verbal act but it also involved activities in everyday situations. Engaging in occupations is an important source of images and acted meanings that can later take verbal forms (Alsaker & Josephsson, 2010).

Asking questions in fieldwork settings differs from interviewing settings. In fieldwork, the questions are tuned into situations that evolve. The researcher takes part in the actual situations that make up the material for acted stories of interest for the analysis. When invited to participate in an activity with the respondent, the situation is used to prompt the respondents along with the occupations that are being shared. Usually, it works well to use the same questions, as the above interview examples, but prompts can be added, for example, "please show me how you did that one more time" or "please teach me how to do this?" Throughout the situations taken part in, questions are asked that are embedded in the context, such as, "have you been to this mall before, is this the mall where you usually do your shopping?"

As a participant observer, it is important to be conscious of positioning or how you choose to act. One potential position is to be a learner, a guest or someone who is new to this situation, something that will provide ways to communicate easily in the situation. A position needs to be chosen, which one is comfortable with as a researcher. Occupational scientists and occupational therapists are usually skilled to observe and participate in everyday occupations alongside people, something that might make this approach to data collection relaxed and enable access to vivid and rich narrative material.

It is challenging to record material in fieldwork settings; therefore, extensive field notes need to be written on completing the observation. Field notes can be described as the accounts describing experiences and observations the researcher has made while participating in an involved manner (Hammersley & Atkinson, 2007). It is important that recorded field notes are rich enough to give grounding for narrative analysis.

Narrative data have, per definition, a social dimension, which means that the researcher will always be part of the generated data. Lawlor and Mattingly (2001) have made useful reflections in this matter arguing that the meaning of relationship as lived experience cannot be studied without being part of the relationship and relating within it. Given that narrative meaning involves emplotting, the argument is particularly relevant when using narrative as research tool. In our study of women living with chronic rheumatic conditions and their engagement in everyday occupations, we particularly reflected on our professional identities which included being occupational therapists. We then needed to consider how possible therapy lenses influenced the analytic process.

Data analysis

In a narrative analysis one builds on how narrative theory is identifying the construction of meaning. Therefore identifying plots and storylines in the data is central to storied analysis. One useful analytical resource in narrative analysis is developed within hermeneutic theory. Hermeneutic theory addresses interpretation and the functions and practices of interpretation (Kaspersen, 2000; Lindseth & Norberg, 2004; Silverman, 2001). Interpretation can be defined as the assignment of possible meanings to situations or language. Further, in hermeneutics, interpretation is identified as a communicative movement between interpretations and the material that makes up the interpretations (a movement often referred to as the hermeneutic circle). We argue that narrative analysis as presented in this chapter is fundamentally hermeneutic.

In line with hermeneutic reasoning, the interpretive activity of narrative analysis involves key characteristics. Analysis needs to be iterative and evolving, moving between possible emplotments that can be created from the material as well as between the emerging emplotments and the material. In order to do this, it is often useful to involve several researchers who can create an interpretative space together for testing, working with, rejecting, and searching for possible plots that will uncover meaning that resonate with the focus of the study. An entrance to find plots to work with can be the significant events that Mattingly (1998) identified as central for narrative meaning-making. A significant event, according to Mattingly, can be seen as part of a story that stands out for the person doing the narration, often central in the structuring of a story.

In the analytical process, an active stance regarding how the analysis will deal with existing theory on the subject understudy is required. It can be very fruitful to set the emerging analysis in dialog with theory, given that a body of knowledge exists. However, this is not the same as using the data to illustrate existing concepts or theory (Polkinghorne, 1995, 2000). Rather, theory is brought into the dialectic move between interpretations and material that characterize hermeneutical interpretation. In hermeneutics, the importance of pre-understandings is identified as central in interpretation. Pre-understandings are the understandings a researcher brings to the reading of a situation or to an emplotment of possible meanings in research. To reflexively bring the pre-understandings to the fore and make explicit when doing narrative research makes the findings more transparent and is an element in establishing trustworthiness of the research.

In the following section, we will give an example of how the analytical activities of a narrative study might unfold based on our study on how meaning in everyday activities is established and revised among women living with chronic health conditions (Alsaker & Josephsson, 2011).

Textbox 6.2 Lily's narrative

Lily is a 53-year-old woman. She has had a severe rheumatic disease since youth, affecting her body and making her dependent on daily medication. She experiences recurrent pain and stiffness in her joints and muscle tissues as well as fatigue. She manages her everyday life, in which she participates in a wide range of activities. This particular day she was about to do some errands together with Sissel.

Driving to town, Lily talked about her need to find a parking space wide enough so that she could open the door of the car completely, because she needed more space than was normal to get out due to her limited range of body movement. She looked for a space in the regular parking areas, as she said that the lots designated for disabled people were either occupied or too narrow for her needs, and that she thought they were mainly for people with wheelchairs or walkers. Finding a parking space with an open space on the driver's side, we got out and strolled along the pavement. Before we left the car she removed her disability parking sign from the car window. After a 10-minute stroll, we reached our goal, an office where she was to deliver something. When this task was completed, we walked back towards the car. Approaching the parked car Lily halted and said, 'You can understand my problems because you are with me for longer periods and do things together with me, but others see me as normal when I am walking down the street. You see, this is about the distance I can walk without slowing down or starting to limp'.

In Textbox 6.2, we present a narrative compiled from the field notes taken during participant observation in our study. Lily is one among a large number of women living with chronic rheumatic conditions around the world. For these persons, personal care, preparing food, and other everyday acts comprising their habitual daily routine are hard to perform. Lily's story is an outcome of the analysis and brings the reader into an everyday situation that appears as though it comes directly from the field notes. However, in the original field notes a description of the actual event was present, that is Lily's parking and walk to her errand and the dialog she had with the researcher. When reading through the field notes and in the reflective notes from the researcher, this situation stood out as being of interest in relation to the aim of the study and thus having qualities that matched with what Mattingly (1998) identified as a significant event. It stood out from the other data by involving some suspense (Lily taking away the disability sign) and riddle (why did she do that?).

The analysis involved some distinctive features that were carried out in an iterative manner in line with hermeneutical interpretation; but it needs to be noted that these were not carried out in a linear manner and thus we present them as inter-twined phases. One phase involved finding the storied structures of the story. In this phase, we developed the event of finding a parking space (as in Textbox 6.2). This was done by working with a large amount of data and identifying how to present a possible story organized around plots. Another phase involved trying out possible emplotments of the story. There were of course several possibilities on how this story could be understood, and this phase involved trying out and testing each possibility. Yet another phase involved setting the evolving emplotments in communication with existing knowledge and theory. In our study, this phase involved theory on living with chronic conditions as well as theory on mean-ing. A central activity in hermeneutical interpretation is the exploring movement between emerging interpretations and data as well as existing theory.

Through the narrative analyses we were able to show, through situated inter-pretation drawing on narrative theory, how the individual (Lily) was navigating between opposites, her available cultural resources (medicine), and her own wish to be and act like everyone else, thereby showing the complexity in unfolding situations. The disability sign could be used and it could be taken away pending the situation. We were also able to see how this move between different images of whom one is involved dilemmas for Lily. Staying in tune with society's as well as the local cultural norms for normality (such as walking without limping or a visible aid) might cause pain or just not be possible because of Lily's pre-sent functioning. However, for a shorter period and if the environment is right, it might be possible to be in tune with the expectation of society and be like others. The analysis showed how the meanings of the everyday actions of Lily played and interacted with the meanings her diagnosis gave. In this way, the narrative analysis was able to uncover how there were multiple dynamic meanings of situ-ations which involved both being able to move in and out of being labeled "dif-ferent". However, this required a lot of effort and planning from Lily's side and further was not always possible. Being placed in situations where she had to work hard and adjust her actions to be like others was also demanding and potentially involved physical pain for Lily.

As demonstrated in the example of Lily, narrative analysis results in analytical possibilities outlining different meanings (or emplotments) of the situations and the meanings researched. In this way, the methodology succeeds in giving access to multiple and moving dimensions of meaning and moves beyond mere descrip-tion. Since narrative methodology gives access to situated shifting knowledge outlining possibilities rather than objective truths, this needs to be communicated when reporting the study. It also puts demands on the researcher to ground analytical procedures in rigorous exploration of analytical possibilities and to make these visible in reporting. These groundings can involve dialogs with informants bringing them into the iterative work with possible emplotments and how these interplay.

In many qualitative methodologies, it is recommended to include several participants and analysis means identifying general themes that are based in all data. However, a central question pertaining to narrative inquiry is whether this form of qualitative inquiry is applicable to data materials including several persons or if it is a methodology applicable to individuals? There is an inherent conflict in this question. As soon as a larger group of informants is included and the analysis needs to account for all data, there is a risk that findings become more generic and thus, to a lesser extent, capture the richness and complexity of the meanings available in the material. At the same time given the social character of meaning-making, we believe that it would be limiting to only use narrative methodology on individual data. The researcher has to resolve the tension between finding the commonalities in the stories while preserving the integrity of the individual narrative.

Presenting findings

Qualitative inquiry often presents findings in form of themes summarizing the key findings of the analysis and grounding these findings in the empirical material with assistance from direct quotes and vignettes from data. This way of structuring the findings has advantages since it gives the reader of the study tools to grasp the key findings and follow the reasoning and groundings of these and the analytical procedures. However, it tends to summarize the findings into general language, thus failing to portray the multitude as well as the moving character of meanings. Therefore, narrative inquiry traditionally presents the material in the form of emerging stories, including several alternative meanings that can be identified from the analysis and the tensions and dialogs that can be seen within and between these interpretations. The stories presented are, however, not taken directly from data. Rather they are the result of the analytical process and constructed to give access to layers of meanings that connect to the focus of the study.

Our study of women living with chronic rheumatic conditions and their engagement in everyday occupations was based on four women's everyday lives. In the findings section, we presented the emplotments resulting from the analysis supported by vignettes that grounded and situated these emplotments in stories stemming from data.

Rigor/ethics

The iterative process of working with possible plots needs time. The trustworthiness of narrative research is dependent on the researchers allowing time for testing and playing with multiple possibilities that are available for interpretations.

Further, analysis requires the ability to keep multiple interpretations and emplotments at play so that the result that is slowly built up resonates with the multifold character of human meaning. Rigor might not be the best term though for interpretative analysis given that it might imply a standard or "true" way of conducting narrative analysis. That said we want to stress the importance of grounding the analysis in iterative communication between data and emerging interpretations to establish quality in the analysis. One strategy to employ is to join with experienced researchers and set the evolving results in dialog with others' interpretations concerns and views. The quality of the result is related to the extent that researchers have been able to explore and try out possibilities of analysis from the existing material.

Engaging with participants over time is a strategy to ensure rigor; however, entering into the lives of participants raises ethical issues. The aim of the researcher is to gather stories which provide a rich understanding of the participant's life and will potentially add to knowledge or influence practice. While ethics committees consider the potential of research causing harm to participants, and researchers have to ensure that the risk of harm is minimized, the participants do not directly benefit from participating in the study. Researchers need to employ reflexivity to consider the impact of the data collection on participant's lives, but more to consider the impact of the relationship that is formed during data collection that is unlikely to be maintained following completion of the study. Each researcher will need to seek his or her own level of comfort around that issue which may depend on the length of engagement and the sensitivity of the topic under exploration.

Critiquing narrative studies

We have already argued that narrative is a very broad concept that depending on the theoretical underpinnings might be rather different endeavors. It is therefore hard to interpret the findings of a narrative study if the theoretical resources are not made explicit. Another trap for the novice is that the analysis is more a representative of the existing theory than an exploration of the area under study. A set of questions to assist with the critique of narrative studies is presented in Textbox 6.3.

Textbox 6.3   Critiquing narrative studies – questions to ask

1   How is the *epistemology* presented and communicated?
2   How is the narrative methodology *grounded in theory*?
3   How is the research question *linked to meanings* of occupational engagement?
4   Does the method section contain detail on how the researchers conducted analysis?
5   How does the evolving and multifaceted character of the findings become apparent?

Application to occupational science

Bonsall (2012) has provided a possible typology of the use of narrative in occupational science drawing on an analysis of journal articles from occupational therapy and occupational science. His third category of research methodology identifies four subcategories of thematic analysis, life histories, narrative slope, and analysis of action. He argued that the typology provides clarity of the usage of narrative to strengthen occupational science research. Moreover, the analysis revealed the study of narratives in relation to life-changing illness or disability and the need for utilizing narrative to understand occupation in a more general sense to add to occupational science knowledge about the importance of occupation.

At the beginning of this chapter, we situated narrative methodology in a current discussion on the need for methodology capable to give access to the situated and unfolding character of occupation. We argued that the current practice of qualitative research might not fully portray the situated and unfolding quality of human occupation. Therefore, we need to develop methodology capable of incorporating these features of human occupation (Alsaker, Josephsson, & Dickie, 2013). We foresee that this move will lead to further methodological developments and shifts in the future.

Application to occupational therapy

Narrative is used within occupational therapy research and occupational therapy practice in a number of ways. Clouston (2003) identified the narrative forms of life histories and life stories, illness narratives, volitional narratives, and occupational narratives. Narrative is used in practice to elicit client stories to better understand the client experience within his or her context. Findings from studies using narrative methodology provides occupational therapists with a deeper understanding of the meaning-making in people's lives as they orchestrate everyday occupations in the context of illness or disability.

Personal reflections

In the beginning of this chapter, we stated our ambition to present narrative methodology as a tool to access unfolding and situated meaning in occupation. We placed narrative methodology in relation to recent calls for qualitative inquiry sensitive to unfolding character of occupations. We had been concerned about how qualitative methodology can make an issue or area less relevant and compelling by twisting the life situations that are often overwhelming and contradictive to structures that are more in line with professional language and perspectives. When we were first introduced to narrative methodology by Cheryl Mattingly in the early 1990s, we became hopeful for a methodology that has a character of ongoing critique and investigation. Narrative methodology can play a part in establishing such sensitizing practice of qualitative methods.

Our current interest is in exploring the basic moral dimension in narrative reasoning (Alsaker & Josephsson, 2011) where moral is understood as the messages conveyed or lessons to be learned from a story, lived or told. One core element in processes of human meaning-making is to get access to, and tools to elaborate on, different moral quests that are present in everyday life. The capacity to address the moral issues embedded in everyday activities is another feature of narrative that corresponds to the concerns raised on contemporary qualitative methods for resulting mainly in descriptive knowledge. The moral dimension taps in to the worlds of situated evolving meaning and makes narrative research endeavor resonate in midst of the evolving stories that make up human life and meaning.

Conclusion

In this chapter, we have described how narrative methodology, while broadly referring to research associated with story-telling, can refer to a broad range of traditions and approaches. Drawing on our own work of narrative in action with women living with chronic rheumatoid disease, we have shown how narrative methodology enables access to the underlying meaning-making involved in human occupation situated in the everyday.

References

Alsaker, S., Bongaardt, R., & Josephsson, S. (2009). Studying narrative-in-action in women with chronic rheumatic conditions. *Qualitative Health Research, 19*(8), 1154–1161. doi:10.1177/1049732309341478.

Alsaker, S., & Josephsson, S. (2010). Occupation and meaning: Narrative in everyday activities of women with chronic rheumatic conditions. *OTJR – Occupation, Participation and Health, 30*(2), 58–67. doi:10.3928/15394492–20100312–01.

Alsaker, S., & Josephsson, S. (2011). Stories stirring the quest of the 'good': Narratives of women living with chronic rheumatic conditions. *Scandinavian Journal of Disability Research, 13*(1), 53–70. doi:10.1080/15017411003711809.

Alsaker, S., Josephsson, S., & Dickie, V. (2013). Exporing the transactional quality of occupations by using narrative-in-action. In V. A. Dickie & M. P. Cutchin (Eds.), *Transactional perspectives on occupation* (pp. 65–77). New York, NY: Springer.

Aristotle. (1920). *Aristotle on the art of poetry.* New York, NY: Oxford University Press.

Bonsall, A. (2012). An examination of the pairing between narrative and occupational science. *Scandinavian Journal of Occupational Therapy, 19*, 92–103.

Bonsall, A. (2013). Fathering occupations: An analysis of narrative accounts of fathering children with special needs. *Journal of Occupational Science.* doi:10.1080/14427591. 2012.760423.

Borell, L., Nygård, L., Asaba, E., Gustavsson, A., & Hemmingson, H. (2012). Qualitative approaches in qualitative research. *Scandinavian Journal of Occupational Therapy, 19*(6), 521–529. doi:10.3109/11038128.2011.649782.

Clouston, T. (2003). Narrative methods: Talk, listening and representation. *British Journal of Occupational Therapy, 66*(4), 136–142.

Denzin, N. K. (2013). "The death of data?" *Cultural Studies ↔ Critical Methodologies, 13*(4), 353–356. doi:10.1177/1532708613487882.

DePoy, E., & Gitlin, L. N. (2011). *Introduction to research* (3rd ed.). St. Louis, MO: Elsevier.

Frank, G., & Polkinghorne, D. (2010). Qualitative research in occupational therapy: From the first to the second generation. *OTJR: Occupation, Participation & Health, 30*(2), 51–57. doi:10.3928/15394492-20100325-02.

Geertz, C. (1973). *The interpretation of cultures.* New York, NY: Basic Books.

Hammersley, M., & Atkinson, P. (2007). *Ethnography: Principles in practice* (3rd ed.). London, UK: Routledge.

Hewitt, A., Howie, L., Feldman, S. (2010). Retirement: What will you do? A narrative inquiry of occupation-based planning for retirement: Implications for practice. *Australian Occupational Therapy Journal, 57,* 8–16. doi:10.111/j.1440–1630.2009.00820.x.

Holstein, J., & Gubrium, J. (2012). *Varieties of narrative analysis.* Los Angeles, CA: Sage.

Josephsson, S., Asaba, E., Jonsson, H., & Alsaker, S. (2006). Creativity and order in communication: Implications from philosophy to narrative research concerning human occupation. *Scandinavian Journal of Occupational Therapy, 13*(2), 125–132.

Josephsson, S., la Cour, K., & Jonsson, H. (2007). Possibility spaces in everyday life: On creative potentials in interventions for persons with life-threatening incurable illness. In C. Dumont & G. Kielhofner (Eds.), *Positive approaches to health* (pp. 37–46). New York, NY: Nova Science Publishers.

Kaspersen, L. B. (2000). *Anthony Giddens – Introduksjon til en samfundsteoretiker* (Anthony Giddens – introduction) (4th ed.). Copenhagen, Denmark: Hans Reitzels Forlag.

Lawlor, M., & Mattingly, C. (2001). Beyond the unobtrusive observer: Reflections on researcher-informant relationships in urban ethnography. *American Journal of Occupational Therapy, 55*(2), 147–154. doi:10.5014/ajot.55.2.147.

Lindseth, A., & Norberg, A. (2004). A phenomenological hermeneutical method for researching lived experience. *Scandinavian Journal of Caring Sciences, 18*(2), 145–153.

Mattingly, C. (1998). *Healing dramas and clinical plots. The narrative structure of experience.* Los Angeles, CA: University of California Press.

Polkinghorne, D. (1995). Narrative configuration in qualitative analyses. *Qualitative Studies in Education, 8*(1), 5–23. doi:10/1080/0951839950080103.

Polkinghorne, D. (2000). Psychological inquiry and the pragmatic and hermeneutic traditions. *Theory & Psychology, 10*(4), 453–479. doi:10.1177/0959354300104002

Ricoeur, P. (1984a). *Time and narrative* (Vol. I–III). Chicago: The University of Chicago Press.

Ricoeur, P. (1984b). *Time and narrative* (Vol. I). Chicago: The University of Chicago Press.

Ricoeur, P. (1991). *From text to action: Essays in hermeneutics.* Evanston, IL: Northwestern University Press.

Silverman, D. (2001). *Interpreting qualitativedata. Methods for analysing talk, text and interaction.* London, UK: Sage.

Stamm, T., Lovelock, L., Stew, G., Nell, V., Snyden, J., Machold, K., . . . Sadlo, G. (2009). I have a disease but I am not ill: A narrative study of occupational balance in people with rheumatoid arthritis. *OTJR Occupation, Participation and Health, 29*(1), 32–39.

Wright-St Clair, V. (2003). Storymaking and storytelling: Making sense of living with multiple sclerosis. *Journal of Occupational Science, 10*(1), 46–51. doi:10.1080/14427591.2003.9686510.

Further reading

Clandinin, J. D. (2007). *Handbook of narrative inquiry: Mapping a methodology.* Los Angeles, CA: Sage.

Wells, K. (2011). *Narrative inquiry.* New York, NY: Oxford University Press.

Website

http://www.methods.manchester.ac.uk/methods/narrative/

7   Ethnography

Understanding occupation through an examination of culture

Suzanne Huot

Ethnography is the study of a group or culture. One of the oldest qualitative methodologies, with roots dating back to the late 1800s and early 1900s, ethnography is often not a well understood methodology. In this chapter, I explain ethnographic methodology and its fit for the study of human occupation. In doing so, I draw upon examples from a critical ethnography I conducted that explored the experiences of French-speaking immigrants from visible minority groups settling in a mid-sized Canadian city.

Drawing on the work of others, Bryman (2001) has provided a comprehensive definition of ethnography that highlights five key features of the approach. First, researchers must immerse themselves in the society or group they are interested in studying. Second, by engaging in fieldwork, researchers collect descriptive data. Third, the data collected must reflect the culture of those being studied. Fourth, the perspective of the research participants and the meanings they attach to their social worlds must be at the center. Finally, findings must be made relevant for target audiences.

There are a diverse range of approaches to ethnography, possibly contributing to the confusion regarding what ethnography 'really is'. Given the array of ethnographic methodologies (e.g., critical ethnography, feminist ethnography, focused ethnography, institutional ethnography, etc.), this chapter will address ethnographic research as a broad school of inquiry characterized by particular features that distinguish it from other methodologies. Within this ethnographic school of inquiry, particular methodological styles may be adopted depending on the purpose of specific research studies. Auto-ethnography will, however, be specifically discussed given its unique focus on the researcher as a study participant.

While still confined within the occupation-focused literature, examples of published ethnographic work include my own research (Huot, Laliberte Rudman, Dodson, & Magalhães, 2013), as well as a range of studies examining diverse topics (e.g. Dickie, 2003; Horghagen & Josephsson, 2010; Peralta-Catipon, 2009; Riley, 2008, 2011); for example, Aldrich and Callanan's (2011) ethnographic study of discouraged workers in rural North Carolina, USA. Ethnography is particularly well suited to studying occupation focusing on everyday lived experiences and the contexts within which these are embedded.

Background

Modern ethnography is typically traced back to traditions within social and cultural anthropology and sociology. Within anthropology, ethnographic origins are largely associated with Malinowski's (1922) seminal fieldwork in the Trobriand Islands, which reflected the perceived need during the early twentieth century for trained ethnographers to undertake primary research, rather than draw upon reports of others, such as colonial travelers. Within sociology, the emergence of ethnography is linked to the Chicago School of the early 1900s. The different disciplinary approaches originating in Britain and the United States provide the foundation for the varying traditions present within this school of inquiry (Bryman, 2001).

As the examination of the culture a group of people share, ethnography provides a close study of that culture according to particular people, places, occupations, and times (Van Maanen, 2004). A focus on the particularities of a lived culture is taken up in ethnographic research to question received truths and to explore whether a perceived societal consensus actually exists or whether dominant hegemonic discourses instead give the appearance of consensus. Despite the challenges of examining current cultures that are characterized by multiple and diverse layers and ethnicities, ethnography provides the opportunity to study participants' historically and socially situated experiences (Lecompte, 2002).

Ethnography is appropriate for examining how people construct their realities within particular social contexts, because it views communities as a collection of individuals rather than monoliths whose "often contentious interactions constitute the fabric of a culture full of hitherto unnoticed diversity" (Lecompte, 2002, p. 292). This is particularly useful for examining people's engagement in daily occupations and considering how their 'doing, being, becoming and belonging' (Whalley Hammell, 2004) are shaped by and serve to reproduce culture.

Epistemology

Early ethnographies were situated within a positivist paradigm, but contemporary ethnographic studies have been expanded through the adoption of contructivist, interpretivist, and critically theoretical paradigm positions. This chapter focuses primarily on research located within these latter paradigms that are viewed as alternatives to positivism because they are more ontologically relativist and acknowledge the existence of multiple realities experienced by diverse populations (Guba & Lincoln, 2004). Understanding of research participants' experiences and occupations are developed in relation to their context through fieldwork and other forms of data collection. Findings generated are located within the relevant current and historical social contexts and analyzed in relation to these contexts.

Epistemologically, data are transactional, intersubjective, and value-mediated. Knowledge is understood as co-constructed through interactions between researcher and participants (Lincoln & Guba, 2003). Viewing knowledge in this way leads to the adoption of dialogical methods to overcome misapprehensions and to promote more informed understanding between the parties involved. The role of the researcher is vital to address through ongoing reflexivity, as "what can be known is inextricably intertwined with the interaction between a *particular* investigator and a *particular* object or group" (Guba & Lincoln, 2004, p. 26).

Auto-ethnography

Auto-ethnography refers to an autobiographical approach to conducting and disseminating research (Bryman, 2001). The study may have a single participant, the researcher, or the researcher's experiences and biography can be included as part of a broader ethnographic work. As the purpose of this methodology is to understand the relationship between individuals and their cultural contexts, using an auto-ethnographic approach has been described as using the self "as a mechanism for weaving back and forth between personal experience and culture" (Bryman, 2001, p. xxxii). Similarly, Hamilton, Smith, and Worthington (2008) described auto-ethnography as bringing forward changing aspects of the self and creating ways to write about one's experiences within a broader social context. Hence, this approach involves self-reflexive ways of knowing and, like other ethnographic methodologies, must follow rigorous research practices (Hamilton et al., 2008).

Defining the topic

Ethnographic research is largely inductive making it well suited to studies of cultures and groups about which additional knowledge is needed. Culture in this sense is not synonymous with ethnicity. Instead, culture should be interpreted broadly as the "acquired knowledge that people use to interpret their world and generate social behavior" (Spradley & McCurdy, 1984, p. 2). Hallmarks of ethnographic research include prolonged engagement and participant observation, whereby researchers immerse themselves in fieldwork by entering naturalistic settings where the group of interest is located. This can include varied environments depending on the research focus, for example, the culture of a group of health professionals in a particular hospital unit, residents living in an assisted care facility, or women in a craft guild.

My research centered on the Francophone minority community (FMC) in London, Ontario. Canada has two official languages, but the majority of the national population is Anglophone. French speakers are mainly located within the province of Quebec, and geographic regions outside of this province that have concentrations of Francophones are designated as FMCs. Over 40% of French-speaking immigrants within the province arrived after 1996, and a large proportion of them came from Africa (Fédération des communautés francophones etacadienne du Canada, 2009). Immigration generates demographic, social, and cultural change within communities. Given the changes occurring within the city's FMC, my ethnography focused on the integration experiences of French-speaking immigrants from visible minority groups living in London. As a Francophone who has lived my entire life within a FMC, this research was particularly important to me. I am a married, Caucasian female in my thirties who was born and raised in Southern Ontario. Having never personally migrated, I have long been interested in people's experiences of international mobility. This study allowed me to meld my Francophone identity with my research interests in migration and enabled me to become an engaged member of the local French-speaking community.

My research objectives were worded to reflect the critical positioning of the ethnography. The first objective was to critically examine the experiences of French-speaking migrants from visible minority groups to challenge unspoken assumptions embedded within notions of 'successful integration' as identified within government documents. The second objective was to raise awareness of the structural barriers these migrants faced in enacting occupation and negotiating their identities within the places they frequented, particularly according to the markers of language, race, and gender. As ethnographies focus on the culture a group of people share, they address the contexts within which groups of individuals are embedded. Research questions, problems, and objectives are worded to address what is happening within the research field of interest (e.g., classroom, rehabilitation center) and why it is happening. This approach enables emphasis to be placed on contextual images and patterns (e.g. values, symbols, norms, beliefs) within the field or site. As described by Van Maanen (2004), ethnography is "the close study of culture as lived by particular people, in particular places, doing particular things at particular times" (p. 440) and is therefore sociohistorically specific.

A key consideration when designing an ethnographic study is how the research field will be defined. The research field is not simply an objective pre-existing space entered from the outside by researchers; it is instead defined by researchers in relation to their objectives (Nast, 1994). This relates, in part, to how the cultural group being studied is defined. Contemporary understandings of culture recognize that it is dynamic rather than static and unchanging. As processes of globalization have accelerated, populations have become less homogenous making it increasingly difficult to study isolated groups within or outside one's own society. Ethnography can thus be used to examine how culture is lived, produced, and reproduced; and from an occupational perspective, explore how the process of cultural change influences, and is influenced by, occupation.

Boundary setting

Key to boundary setting is defining the population being studied and identifying the site(s) where fieldwork will occur. I chose to study the experiences of Francophone immigrants from visible minority groups. 'Francophone' was defined as people whose mother tongue or first official language is French. 'Immigrants' was used broadly to include all classes and categories of immigrants as well as refugees and asylum seekers. 'Visible minority groups' was not strictly defined, allowing research participants to self-identify. I chose to focus on London because it is a designated FMC within Southwestern Ontario, a geographic region that has been understudied in the literature on Francophone immigration to Canada.

Once the group and field of interest are defined, and institutional ethics approval is obtained, participants can be recruited. Recruitment in ethnographic research should be purposeful to achieve a depth of understanding. Successful recruitment is dependent on access to the cultural group and entry into the field. This can be achieved using different techniques. For instance, a gatekeeper who knows members of the group can be approached to assist with recruitment. Standard techniques for recruitment such as the dissemination of study information can also be used, but may not generate the most purposeful group of participants.

Recruitment

Within my study, I used a range of strategies to gain entry into the field. Potential strategies, including those I used, are summarized in Textbox 7.1.

Textbox 7.1   Entering the field – potential strategies

1   Use the Internet to explore what organizations, services, and programs are available within the community
2   Arrange meetings with contacts from community organizations to discuss research
3   Regularly attend community events, festivals, meetings, and forums
4   Volunteer for community organizations and programs
5   Get involved with community initiatives

I recruited two different participant groups. The first group reflected the main population of interest: French-speaking immigrants from visible minority groups residing in London. As I aimed to explore the interrelationships between this group and the broader social locale within which they were embedded, I recruited a second group of participants who could provide details regarding the socio-historical context: employees or members of the boards of directors from local government and nonprofit organizations. The first group included both women and men to allow a gender-based analysis. Participants had to have immigrated to Canada from another country, be French-speaking adults between 18 and 65 years of age, and self-identify as members of visible minority groups. I also sought participants who had been in London for varying lengths of time to provide insight into the dimensions of integration that occur over a number of years. For the second group, I sought men and women employees, members of the board or directors, or representatives of governmental and nonprofit organizations geared toward immigrant settlement and integration within the community. Snowball sampling occurred as respondents suggested additional contacts.

Participants in both groups were recruited through a variety of means. I had made contacts within the community before beginning formal data collection. A gatekeeper in one of the community organizations forwarded a recruitment advertisement via email to the organization's contact list, which consisted largely of immigrant clients using the center's settlement services. I also left hard copies of the advertisement and letters of information in the reception area of two community organizations that provide services to immigrants. This initial strategy led to five responses within 1 month. Reflecting the iterative nature of ethnography, additional recruitment was withheld to allow for preliminary data generation and analysis so that further recruitment could be purposefully informed by emerging insights. Once data generation with this initial group was nearing completion, I sought to recruit additional participants. Recruitment took a more targeted approach using word-of-mouth or 'snowball' approach to purposefully locate people who could provide additional insight. For instance, the initial respondents were mostly male and I wanted to understand the gendered nature of the integration process, requiring the targeted recruitment of female participants.

Participants in the second group were recruited mainly through personal communication. Having begun my immersion into the field during the year prior to beginning formal data collection (e.g., attending community events, volunteering for organizations), I was becoming increasingly known within the FMC, which facilitated recruitment. There is no standard for the number of participants that should be included in an ethnographic study. The decision to stop recruiting should be informed by a number of considerations, including the approaches to data collection selected (e.g., the range of methods used, the number of sessions conducted), practical constraints (e.g., time and resources), and success in identifying information rich participants, among others. Across the two groups, I recruited 14 participants in total, and given my methodological approach and variety of methods used, I engaged in 43 individual data collection sessions. This resulted in a large volume of rich textual, observational, and visual data.

Data collection methods

Within ethnographic research, a variety of methods may be utilized. I used a critical ethnographic approach adapted from Carspecken (1996) to design my study and select my data collection methods.

An ethnographic approach is intended to study action occurring within social sites and to understand that action by exploring the locales and social systems within which those sites are embedded. It is "designed to assess the subjective experiences common to actors on the site and to determine the significance of the activities" (Carspecken, 1996, p. 40) *in relation* to the larger social system. The social system is not understood as existing separately from human activity; rather it is comprised by patterned human activity, meaning that its existence depends on its continual reproduction. Carspecken's work is located within educational research, but his approach has been used in research with migrants (Naidoo, 2008). Although I adapted the approach to suit the focus of my study, the overall design is coherent with his emphasis on a process of dialogical data generation through interviews and observations, as well as the inclusion of secondary data to enable an examination of the relationship between the sites where research occurs and their location within the broader social structure. I engaged in five stages of

Table 7.1 The five stages of critical ethnographic data generation and analysis

Stage	Data generation and analysis
1	Narrative interviews (one session)
2	'Occupational mapping' and participatory occupations (two sessions)
3	In-depth interviews (two sessions)
4	Document analysis and in-depth interviews with representatives from governmental and nonprofit organizations (one session)
5	Data analysis and interpretation

data generation and analysis presented in Table 7.1. These stages resulted in five individual data collection sessions with each participant in the first group (i.e., stages one through three) and one session with each participant in the second group (i.e., stage four).

Narrative and in-depth interviews

I conducted three interviews with each of the eight French-speaking immigrants from visible minority groups: an initial narrative-style interview (stage one) and two in-depth interviews (stage three). As the participants came to London from different countries, I was not familiar with the context of their migration and the narrative interview sensitized me to their experiences. I used the following prompt, based on Wengraf's (2001) approach to lightly structured narrative interviewing, to collect their stories: "Tell me the story of your experience of international migration, and what your experience of coming to, and living in, London has been like?" Participants shared their story of migration, settlement, and integration in as much or as little detail as they wished to emphasize the issues that were important to them.

The subsequent in-depth interviews were initially developed to address the research objectives and were loosely separated into the broad categories of 'occupation' and 'integration' focused questions (e.g., Tell me about what a typical day is like for you. What helped or hindered your migration experience?). These sessions served to further supplement and clarify information collected during earlier stages by providing an opportunity to ask follow-up questions. For instance, the Muslim female respondent emphasized how wearing a niqab led some people to falsely assume that she could not do particular things, such as obtain a drivers license. To explore this occupational issue further, I asked her to share additional examples and she discussed the challenges she faced to labor market integration given how veiled women may be perceived by others:

> You won't find a job. Because you know, when I had an interview at [potential employer], I wasn't alone, there were a lot of candidates with me. I saw, when you compare, why will they choose a woman with all black like that, and it was the position of secretary, receptionist . . . there are others with hair, makeup and all that, why would they choose this?

Issues that were raised by multiple participants served to inform the development of follow-up interview questions to gain additional perspectives, and depth of understanding, regarding particular issues.

To consider the participants' experiences in relation to the broader structure within which they were embedded, I conducted a single in-depth interview with each person from the second group of participants (stage four). Initially, interview questions addressed the organizations' mandates and principle activities, and their relationship with Francophone immigrants. Additional questions were asked throughout the interview, either following on comments that were previously made or to address issues that arose in earlier interviews with other participants. For instance, whether participants felt the community was united or divided was addressed, as comments related to this issue were made during some of the interviews. All interviews, across the four stages, were digitally recorded.

Occupational mapping and participatory occupations

I designed an 'occupational mapping' exercise where participants in the first group were asked to draw and explain their map of London (stage two). This included telling me about the places they went and what occupations they engaged in there. The maps detailed local spatial use and served to identify occupations that participants may not have thought important enough to highlight explicitly during interviews. These sessions were digitally recorded.

Given the occupational focus of my research, I actively engaged in selected meaningful and routine occupations with each of the participants from group one on two separate occasions and referred to these sessions as 'participatory occupations' (stage two). We performed a range of occupations together such as preparing meals, attending church, running errands, going to the hospital, visiting community organizations, spending time with family, and participating in leisure activities. Whenever possible, the participatory occupation sessions were digitally recorded and when recording was not possible (e.g. while riding bicycles) detailed field notes were taken following completion of the session. Descriptions included observations relating to elements such as the setting and details of the occupation performed. For instance, I examined what was occurring in the site and considered what roles the participants were fulfilling (e.g., employee, friend, parent, spouse). Field notes captured comments taken from memory following the period of observation and my reflections. The record was thus a dense and focused account of the participants' occupations, social interactions, places, and activities (Carspecken, 1996).

Document review

To explore how immigration and integration into FMCs is framed by the government, federal and provincial policy documents relevant to this study were examined to better understand the sociohistoric context within which the migrants were embedded (stage four). These documents were located through the Internet with keyword searches and targeted searches on the websites of particular government agencies (e.g., Office of the Commissioner of Official Languages), as well as searching the bibliographies of documents retrieved. Additional hard-copy documentation was obtained at conferences and forums.

Data analysis

Approaches to analysis must be selected for every method used and the types of data collected. The methods I used generated textual, observational, and visual data. The approach I designed for analyzing each of these is outlined below, reflecting Creswell's (1998) assertion that data analysis is not "off-the-shelf; rather, it is custom-built, revised, and choreographed" and "learned by doing" (p. 142). The process outlined contributed to my immersion in the data and served to deepen my understanding of the participants' experiences.

Textual data

Digital recordings of dialogic data generation sessions held with participants in both groups during stages one through four were transcribed verbatim providing one form of textual data. Government documents (stage four) were a second form of textual data.

By transcribing and reading the transcripts individually, I engaged in a process of 'whole-text analysis' (Ryan & Russell Bernard, 2003; Sandelowski, 1995). I identified key threads emphasized by each of the participants and developed a sense of each individual transcript before beginning any comparison.

All transcripts were then entered into NVivo. Using a low-level coding approach (Carspecken, 1996), the initial stage of open coding entailed a line-by-line approach that remains close to the transcript and is not highly abstracted. These initial 'raw' codes (e.g., child care, transportation) were used to include the participants' opinions as they were voiced. Each transcript was coded in its entirety. The process remained iterative and inductive. As analysis was conducted concurrently with ongoing data generation, insights developed over the course of the study served to inform further data generation and analysis.

Following open coding, the transcripts were analyzed using high-level, theoretical codes that required more abstraction and interpretation. All transcripts were again analyzed in full. In this stage, the code was based on more than the transcript alone (Carspecken, 1996), and I applied concepts from the theoretical framework guiding my study (e.g., habitus, occupation, gender). Given that I conducted a *critical* ethnography, findings stem from the data themselves (i.e., 'pure' induction) and from my critically informed analysis and interpretation process.

Once the coding of transcripts was complete, the individual codes were reorganized into categories. Each category was then explored by examining its component codes, and findings were further elaborated following this analysis process.

Document review

As the government documents included for review in the study were not dialogically generated, they were analyzed differently than the data co-constructed with participants. The documents were read in their entirety to obtain a sense of the whole. Many dealt with a range of issues relevant to FMCs (e.g., education, health care), so I isolated the sections of the documents that specifically addressed immigration. These portions of the documents were analyzed to identify recurrent themes. A careful reading enabled my description and interpretation both of what was stressed within the documents (e.g., How was 'integration' defined within them?) and what was absent (e.g., What did definitions of integration fail to consider?). The documents were not merely summarized; they were interrogated and critiqued.

Observational data

Participant observation occurred in multiple sites during my study (e.g., participants' homes, community center). I described the sites within which each formal data collection session took place, and these detailed field notes formed the observation 'record' together with thick descriptions of what took place during the sessions, as well as my reflections about the sessions. The record was read and re-read and served to further develop the interview guides that were used in the following stages. It also served to highlight themes, issues, and areas of inquiry that were addressed in subsequent interviews and emphasized in analyses of the textual data.

Visual data

The occupational maps were first analyzed on their own. Their content was identified and described (e.g., types of places, presence of roads). In addition to exploring what was included on the maps and how things were presented, I also considered what was absent (e.g., presence of large blank spaces on the map in general or absence of specific places such as grocery stores). I then compared and contrasted the maps. The maps were not considered in isolation from other forms of data. The insights drawn from the analysis of textual and observational data informed my understanding of the maps. Likewise, my analysis of the maps contributed to my interpretation of the textual and observational data. This was possible because the different types of data collected enabled participants to address their experiences in a variety of ways.

Findings

The product of ethnographic research is not simply a report of researchers' fieldwork. Bryman (2001) explained that ethnography has increasingly been viewed "as an attempt to persuade an audience of its credibility and importance" (p. xxxvi). This has led to a diversity of dissemination styles. Particular elements present within the findings should address details regarding the researchers' prolonged engagement in the field, how they accessed the population and entered the sites of interest, their exit from the field, and how the voices of participants and researcher are represented within the text (Bryman, 2001).

The researchers' ongoing engagement in reflexivity should also be documented including a discussion of researchers' positionality with respect to the study. For instance, is the researcher an 'insider' or an 'outsider' to the cultural group being studied? In times where this dichotomy is too simplistic, researchers should detail who they are and how this shaped the conduct of the study. These issues reflect important considerations characteristic of the alternative paradigms that aim to understand the multiple realities experienced by research participants, as well as the role of the researcher in co-constructing interpretations of these experiences with them. The presentation of findings should ultimately reflect the ontological and epistemological positioning of the study.

My critical ethnography addressed individual experiences of migration and integration as embedded within a particular sociohistoric context. Individual experiences were emphasized throughout the first three data collection stages. The ways that migration and integration into FMCs are framed by, and are embedded within, the social structure has material implications for the daily lives of immigrants who are affected by the resulting government policies, strategies, and action plans developed to address this issue. The broader context within which immigrants' experiences were embedded was, therefore, highlighted by stage four of the ethnography. Findings that stemmed from the various forms of data collected were integrated to present a comprehensive discussion in response to the research objectives. Illustrative examples from the data were included to support my interpretations, such as direct quotations from interview transcripts and government documents, example maps, and descriptions taken from the observation record.

Data management

The different forms of data collected must all be managed throughout the study. Each session was digitally recorded and I transcribed the recordings verbatim. Each transcript was entered into two separate NVivo projects. One was used for the open coding and another was used for the theoretical coding. Given the volume of codes generated across the two stages of coding, the software was useful for keeping an alphabetical list that could be scrolled through as analysis progressed. Following the completion of analysis, a report was printed for each code created that included all relevant information from each transcript. This facilitated the process of creating categories.

Field notes were typed and kept in a single Word file to enable them to be read in their entirety to inform the ongoing progress of the study. Pseudonyms were also used to identify the occupational maps. These were not reproduced in their entirety for publication as some were very detailed and could potentially identify participants. The maps were narratively described, and sample maps inspired by the originals were included as visual examples. Hard copies of government documents were obtained or printed from electronic versions and kept together to facilitate their analysis.

Rigor and ethics

The rigor of a study is dependent on the type of ethnography being conducted as well as its guiding philosophical principles. As I completed a critical ethnography,

I was guided by Jamal's (2005) argument that a critical ethnography must satisfy three conditions. First, it must be organized in a way that ensures approaches to data collection and analysis are consistent with the study aims. This ensures a coherent approach with a clear connection between the ontological and epistemological positions guiding the work, and the methodology and methods used to carry out the study is established. For instance, the methods of data generation, analysis and interpretation I selected were inductive, theoretically informed, and dialogical to reflect my belief in the co-construction of knowledge.

Second, the work must be conceived as a starting point for changing the conditions of oppressive and unfair regulations. While critical ontology strives to improve the lives of those within vulnerable positions in society, this is done by recognizing that vulnerability is not an individual problem. Instead, people are made powerless by dominant social forces. My work did not seek to 'change' the participants by making them more amenable to existing Canadian society; rather, I sought to learn from their experiences to better understand the challenges and barriers immigrants may face and to convey that understanding to a wider audience.

Third, the work must acknowledge and discuss the limits of its own claims. While the intent of my research was not to produce generalizable findings, insights drawn from the study may be transferable to other FMCs because they highlight the challenges and opportunities faced by a particular group of people. Nonetheless, the dialogical nature of the data generation procedures should be emphasized throughout so that people can locate the research within the particular context in which it was conducted.

In addition to seeking ethics approval from institutional research ethics boards and obtaining informed consent from all participants before beginning research, ethnographic researchers must also attend to 'ethics in practice' (Guillemin & Gillam, 2004). The critical nature of my research raised particular ethical considerations. I had to remain aware of the real and perceived power differentials between myself and the participants, particularly with respect to race. As all participants were members of visible minority groups, I had to be sensitive to the racial connotations of the research. Issues of representation were also important to consider. Research itself can be a colonizing force as people have been inaccurately represented by outsiders throughout history. Therefore, allowing participants to self-identify within this study and enabling them to co-construct the data promoted a form of shared ownership that respected their contribution. Reciprocity was emphasized throughout this research to ensure that the immigrants and the FMC benefited from the time they devoted to participating in the study. This process began through my involvement in various community functions before data generation, continued with opportunities for collaboration throughout the ethnographic study and moves forward with knowledge mobilization strategies that followed its conclusion.

Critiquing ethnographic studies

Particular questions can be asked to assist the critique of ethnographic studies. The questions featured in Textbox 7.2 reflect strategies recommended by Carspecken

(1996) for ensuring methodological quality in ethnography. The application of common techniques to ensure rigor (e.g., member-checking) will vary based on the ontological and epistemological positioning of a study; however, similar techniques are often used.

Textbox 7.2   Critiquing ethnographic studies – questions to ask

1   Did the research use a *flexible observation schedule*?
2   Was *prolonged engagement* practiced with the participants?
3   Were the same participants *interviewed repeatedly*?
4   Were participants encouraged to use and explain the terms they use in *naturalistic contexts*?
5   Did the researcher use a *low-inference vocabulary* and add interpretations later?
6   Were *consistency checks* conducted between observed activity and what was said in interviews?

Application to occupational science

Occupational scientists have increasingly called for studies that attend to how occupation is dialectically related to the context within which it is situated. Recent research integrating social theory into studies of occupation have also begun to critique the emphasis on individualism within the discipline (Dickie, Cutchin, & Humphry, 2006; Laliberte Rudman, Huot, & Dennhardt, 2009; Suto, 2009). My ethnography attends to the situated nature of occupation by considering how individuals' opportunities, or lack thereof, for occupation are mediated by their identities within and across different places. The experiences of the French-speaking immigrants from visible minority groups were explored in relation to the socio-historic context within which Francophone immigration to Canada is currently embedded.

The study participants experienced a number of transitions that they continue to negotiate. While research addressing transitions within occupational science has emphasized the importance of occupational engagement for facilitating the continuity of identity over time, one's need or ability to re-engage in similar occupations following international migration has not been sufficiently problematized. My study addresses how the shift in place, experienced as a result of migration, alters people's possibilities for occupation and hence their identities. The participants' need to engage in new occupations within Canada, or the restrictions they face in engaging in other occupations, highlights how the development of their identities within the host society both informs and is shaped by their occupational possibilities (Laliberte Rudman, 2010). Essentially, migrants' capacity to engage in specific occupations to confirm or reaffirm their identities may be restricted. My research further contributes to the growing number of studies on migration within occupational science that make the implied role of occupation within discussions of immigrant integration more explicit.

Application to occupational therapy

Some ethnographies may have more direct applications to therapeutic practice than others depending on their focus. Ethnographies examining diverse issues are presented within a range of occupational therapy journals. For example, Pickens, O'Reilly, and Sharp (2010) explored the nature of occupations for family caregivers of people in hospice care over a 6-month period. Magasi and Hammel (2009) conducted a 16-month ethnography examining the experiences of living in a nursing home for women with disabilities. Prodinger, Shaw, Laliberte Rudman, and Townsend (2012) critically explored the work of occupational therapists in an outpatient hospital setting for rheumatology using institutional ethnography. Mynard, Howie, and Collister (2009) used ethnography to study a recreational football team geared toward people coping with mental illness, unemployment, addictions, and homelessness over the course of an entire season. These studies each used several data collection approaches including participant observation, interviews, focus groups, and document analysis.

Examining the culture that a particular group of people share can promote culturally safe practice by therapists (National Aboriginal Health Organization, 2008). Global acceleration of international migration has led to increasingly diverse societies. Occupational therapists often have to work with clients whose worldviews, beliefs, values, and norms may differ from their own. To provide holistic, client-centered, and culturally safe care, therapists must recognize that culture is context dependent and is shaped by dominant discourses and social power relations. Ethnographic research is well suited to studies of culture that can provide a broader context for better understanding individual experiences.

Personal reflections

I was initially daunted by the thought of undertaking ethnography. Given the long history and varied traditions characterizing this school of inquiry, I was apprehensive about the decisions that needed to be made to satisfy the hallmarks of this approach. How would I define the cultural group I wanted to study? How would I select the sites where observations could take place? How would I gain access to the community? How long would I have to immerse myself in the field? How would I manage the large amounts of data collected? Despite these initial uncertainties and hesitations, selecting an ethnographic approach was rewarding due to the flexibility it allowed.

This school of inquiry encouraged me to use multiple data collection strategies and to spend an extended period of time with the participants, which promoted a depth of understanding that may not otherwise have been possible. The focus in ethnography on the relationship between individuals and the larger contexts that shape and are reproduced by daily practices was particularly useful for my theoretical interest in bridging the dichotomy between structure and agency. This approach enabled me to examine both the experiences of individual migrants and to explore how these experiences were related to broader contextual factors including governmental immigration policies, eligibility for government-funded services provided by community organizations, and systems of oppression such as racism and sexism, among others. Conducting this study was a truly rewarding experience. Embedded within a larger Anglophone city, I did not often speak my mother tongue. When starting my ethnography, I felt slightly guilty for not having better maintained my language skills. Yet, critically exploring the FMC context led to my increasing awareness of the structural barriers hindering the expression of identities and engagement in occupations for members of minority communities. As noted in the occupation-based literature, identity is not solely something that we are; it is also something that we *do*. Indeed, completing this research was a consciousness raising experience that enabled me to reclaim my Francophone identity, reflecting the aims of critical ethnography to increase awareness of social systems and structures among those involved.

Summary

While maintaining the key characteristics of participant observation, fieldwork, and prolonged engagement, ethnography has greatly evolved from its early beginnings. This has presented new and interesting research opportunities to study a range of groups and cultures (e.g. the culture of an online chat room). The range of methods utilized enable research participants to both 'show and tell' occupation. For occupational scientists and occupational therapists, this school of inquiry and its methodologies support approaches to study how occupations are culturally based and how they are shaped by the broader social context within which engagement takes place.

References

Aldrich, R. M., & Callanan, Y. (2011). Insights about researching discouraged workers. *Journal of Occupational Science, 18*(2), 153–166. doi:10.1080/14427591.2011.575756.

Bryman, A. (2001). Introduction: A review of ethnography. In A. Bryman (Ed.), *Ethnography* (Vol. 1, pp. ix–xxxix). Thousand Oaks, CA: Sage.

Carspecken, P. F. (1996). *Critical ethnography in educational research: A theoretical and practical guide.* New York, NY: Routledge.

Creswell, J. (1998). Data analyses and representation. In J. Creswell (Ed.), *Qualitative inquiry and research design: Choosing among five traditions* (pp. 139–166). Thousand Oaks, CA: Sage.

Dickie, V. A. (2003). The role of learning in quilt making. *Journal of Occupational Science, 10*(3), 120–129. doi:10.1080/14427591.2003.9686519.

Dickie, V. A., Cutchin, M. P., & Humphry, R. (2006). Occupation as transactional experience: A critique of individualism in occupational science. *Journal of Occupational Science, 13*(1), 83–93. doi:10.1080/14427591.2006.9686573.

Fédération des communautés francophones et acadienne du Canada. (2009). *Francophone community profile of Ontario.* Retrieved from http://www.fcfa.ca/profils/documents/ontario_en.pdf

Guba, E. G., & Lincoln, Y. S. (2004). Competing paradigms in qualitative research: Theories and issues. In S. Nagy Hesse-Biber & P. Leavy (Eds.), *Approaches to qualitative research: A reader on theory and practice* (pp. 17–38). Toronto, Canada: Oxford University Press.

Guillemin, M., & Gillam, L. (2004). Ethics, reflexivity, and "ethically important moments" in research. *Qualitative Inquiry, 10*(2), 261–280. doi:10.1177/1077800403262360.

Hamilton, M. L., Smith, L., & Worthington, K. (2008). Fitting the methodology with the research: An exploration of narrative, self-study and auto-ethnography. *Studying Teacher Education, 4*(1), 17–28. doi:10.1080/17425960801976321.

Horghagen, S., & Josephsson, S. (2010). Theatre as liberation, collaboration and relationship for asylum seekers. *Journal of Occupational Science, 17*(3), 168–176. doi: 10.1080/14427591.2010.9686691.

Huot, S., Laliberte Rudman, D., Dodson, B., & Magalhães, L. (2013). Expanding policy-based conceptualizations of 'successful integration': Negotiating integration through occupation following international migration. *Journal of Occupational Science, 20*(1), 6–22. doi:10.1080/14427591.2012.717497.

Jamal, S. (2005). Critical ethnography: An effective way to conduct anti-racism research. In G. J. S. Dei & J. Singh (Eds.), *Critical issues in anti-racist research methodologies* (pp. 225–240). New York, NY: Peter Lang.

Laliberte Rudman, D., Huot, S., & Dennhardt, S. (2009). Shaping ideal places for retirement: Occupational possibilities within contemporary media. *Journal of Occupational Science, 16*(1), 18–24. doi:10.1080/14427591.2009.9686637.

Lecompte, M. (2002). The transformation of ethnographic practice: Past and current challenges. *Qualitative Research, 2*(3), 283–299. doi:10.1177/146879410200200301.

Lincoln, Y. S., & Guba, E. (2003). Paradigmatic controversies, contradictions, and emerging confluences. In N. K. Denzin & Y. S. Lincoln (Eds.), *The landscape of qualitative research* (pp. 253–291). Thousand Oaks, CA: Sage.

Magasi, S., & Hammel, J. (2009). Women with disabilities' experiences in long-term care: A case for social justice. *American Journal of Occupational Therapy, 63*(1), 35–45. doi:http://dx.doi.org/10.5014/ajot.63.1.35.

Malinowski, B. (1922). *Argonauts of the western Pacific: An account of native enterprise and adventure in the archipelagoes of Melanesian New Guinea.* London, UK: Routledge.

Mynard, L., Howie, L., & Collister, L. (2009). Belonging to a community-based football team: An ethnographic study. *Australian Occupational Therapy Journal, 56*(4), 266–274. doi:10.1111/j.1440-1630.2008.00741.x.

Naidoo, L. (2008). Supporting African refugees in Greater Western Sydney: A critical ethnography of after-school homework tutoring centres. *Educational Research for Policy and Practice, 7*(3), 139–150. doi:10.1007/s10671-008-9046-1.

Nast, H. J. (1994). Women in the field: Critical feminist methodologies and theoretical perspectives. *Professional Geographer, 46*(1), 54–66.

National Aboriginal Health Organization. (2008). *Cultural competency and safety: A guide for health care administrators, providers, and educators.* Retrieved from http://www. naho.ca/documents/naho/publications/culturalCompetency.pdf

Peralta-Catipon, T. (2009). Statue square as a liminal sphere: Transforming space and place in migrant adaptation. *Journal of Occupational Science, 16*(1), 32–37.doi:10.108 0/14427591.2009.9686639.

Pickens, N. D., O'Reilly, K. R., & Sharp, K. C. (2010). Holding onto normalcy and overshadowed needs: Family caregiving at end of life. *Canadian Journal of Occupational Therapy, 77*(4), 234–240. doi:http://dx.doi.org/10.2182/cjot.2010.77.4.5.

Prodinger, B., Shaw, L., Laliberte Rudman, D., & Townsend, E. (2012). Arthritis-related occupational therapy: Making invisible ruling relations visible using institutional ethnography. *British Journal of Occupational Therapy, 75*(10), 463–470. doi:http://dx.doi.org/10.4276/030802212X13496921049707.

Riley, J. (2008). Weaving an enhanced sense of self and a collective sense of self through creative textile-making. *Journal of Occupational Science, 15*(2), 63–73. doi:10.1080/14427591.2008.9686611.

Riley, J. (2011). Shaping textile-making: Its occupational forms and domain. *Journal of Occupational Science, 18*(4), 322–338. doi:10.1080/14427591.2011.584518.

Ryan, G. W., & Russell Bernard, H. (2003). Data management and analysis methods. In N. K. Denzin & Y. S. Lincoln (Eds.), *Collecting and interpreting qualitative materials* (pp. 259–309). Thousand Oaks, CA: Sage.

Sandelowski, M. (1995). Qualitative analysis: What is it and how to begin. *Research in Nursing and Health, 18*(4), 371–375. doi:10.1002/nur.4770180411.

Spradley, J. P., & McCurdy, D. W. (1984). *Conformity and conflict: Readings in cultural anthropology.* Toronto, Canada: Little, Brown and Company.

Suto, M. (2009). Compromised careers: The occupational transition of immigration and resettlement. *WORK: A Journal of Prevention, Assessment and Rehabilitation, 32*, 417–429. doi:10.3233/WOR-2009–0853.

Van Maanen, J. (2004). An end to innocence: The ethnography of ethnography. In S. Nagy Hesse-Biber & P. Leavy (Eds.), *Approaches to qualitative research: A reader on theory and practice* (pp. 427–446). Toronto, Canada: Oxford University Press.

Wengraf, T. (2001). *Qualitative research interviewing: Biographic narrative and semi-structured methods.* Thousand Oaks, CA: Sage.

Whalley Hammell, K. (2004). Dimensions of meaning in the occupations of daily life. *Canadian Journal of Occupational Therapy, 71*(5), 296–305.

Further reading

Anderson, G. L. (1989). Critical ethnography in education: Origins, current status, and new directions. *Review of Educational Research, 59*(3), 249–270.

Cook, K. E. (2005). Using critical ethnography to explore issues in health promotion. *Qualitative Health Research, 15*(1), 129–138. doi:10.1177/1049732304267751.

Georgiou, D., & Carspecken, P. F. (2002). Critical ethnography and ecological psychology: Conceptual and empirical explorations of a synthesis. *Qualitative Inquiry, 8*(6), 688–706.

Hardcastle, M., Usher, K., & Holmes, C. (2006). Carspecken's five-stage critical qualitative research method: An application to nursing research. *Qualitative Health Research, 16*(1), 151–161. doi:10.1177/1049732305283998.

Laliberte Rudman, D. (2010). Occupational possibilities. *Journal of Occupational Science, 17*, 55–59.

Stacey, J. (1988). Can there be a feminist ethnography? *Women's Studies International Forum, 11*(1), 115–123.

8 Action research

Exploring occupation and transforming occupational therapy

Clare Wilding and Danika Galvin

Action research, as its name implies, has dual foci of learning and change. With the emphasis on both developing understanding and enacting change, this dynamic form of research is well suited to facilitating the implementation of occupational science concepts and for renewing occupational therapy practice. In this chapter, drawing upon action research studies that we undertook as higher degree students, we will illustrate that action research is a complex, exciting, and powerful methodology for enabling transformative learning and change.

Background and epistemology

Action research is not a singular method; rather it is "a set of theories and principles that guide research" (Klein, 2012, p. 5). It is an approach to research that emphasizes discovery, taking action (Bray, Lee, Smith, & Yorks, 2000) and improving practice (Carr, 2009). Kurt Lewin is credited as the original pioneer of action research in the 1940s (Gustavsen, 2006); however, the philosophical origins of action research are evident in various cultures and social movements worldwide (Reason & Bradbury, 2006). A variety of theoretical viewpoints have influenced the development of action research, including pragmatic philosophy, humanistic philosophy, and complexity theory (Reason & Bradbury, 2006).

A desire to learn lies at the heart of action research (Bray et al., 2000; McNiff & Whitehead, 2010). The learning that is achieved then inspires action to be taken, through which transformation is accomplished. Discovery is attained by "problematizing" an "aspect of one's life-world" (Bray et al., 2000, p. 24). Framing an issue as a problem enables people to explore, question, and become critical of situations that are dominating them; and thus, the "challenging reality" is "unveiled" (Bray et al., 2000, p. 38). Through this confrontation and growing consciousness of an oppressive situation, those who are oppressed are stimulated to transform their world by taking action (Freire, 1970).

As well as learning through problematizing, learning may also be achieved by sharing aspirations about what might produce a better world and by sharing examples of success in achieving the desired situation. Ludema, Cooperrider, and Barrett (2006) advocated for the value of more positive or appreciative forms of action research that can evoke possibilities for imagining and building a better future. Thus, the change achieved in action research aims to be *emancipatory* and may be implicit in the very first questions that a researcher asks (Ludema et al., 2006).

Authentic change cannot be achieved solely through individual forms of empowerment; collective action is also required (Kemmis & McTaggart, 2005). As such, action research is essentially *collaborative* (Bray et al., 2000). A collaborative approach builds new ideas and a supportive network of relationships that can help to maintain research activity over time (Stringer, 2007). Thus, action researchers aspire to manifest learning and change on a grand scale. For example, action researchers may aim to revolutionize individuals and individual practice, or the culture of groups, institutions, and society (Kemmis & McTaggart, 1988).

Collaboration is enhanced by promoting democratic forms of dialog (Gustavsen, 2006). Dialog is important because critical knowledge and self-reflection about tensions, dilemmas, or uncertainties does not automatically translate to knowing what to do to improve the situation (Kemmis, 2006). It is through formation of a public "communicative space" that mutual understanding and consensus about what to do can be developed (Kemmis & McTaggart, 2005, p. 578). Raised consciousness and commitment to action is developed through dialog centered on mutual sharing of wisdom and expertise (Ife, 2008).

Given that action research is emancipatory and collaborative and that it is rooted in overcoming oppression (Freire, 1970), it is not surprising that action research also aspires to be socially just; it is focused on understanding, then changing, and ultimately improving, social situations and social practices (Kemmis & McTaggart, 1988). The purpose of action research is not merely to create change; rather it is to redress the social injustices that have been uncovered and to rectify previous inequalities. Thus, action research facilitates social critique and social action (Townsend, Birch, Langley, & Langille, 2000).

Further, action research is a process that is critically self-reflective (Kemmis & McTaggart, 1988; Koch & Kralik, 2001; Koch, Selim, & Kralik, 2002). The aim of action research is "to plan, act, observe and reflect more carefully, more systematically, and more rigorously than one usually does in everyday life and to use the relationships between these moments in the process as a source of both improvement and knowledge" (Kemmis & McTaggart, 1988, p. 10). The action research process includes challenging taken-for-granted understandings through critical reflection of self and contexts and using this understanding to create opportunities for personal and collective growth and transformation (Cockburn & Trentham, 2002; Soltis-Jarrett, 1997). Through critical questioning, action researchers may become more aware about how their own conceptions of the situation trap them in certain ways of being, thinking, and doing (Gaventa & Cornwall, 2006). Action research is typically enacted as an action research spiral, or cycles of action and reflection (Kemmis & McTaggart, 2005) (Figure 8.1).

Although these cycles of action research are presented in an orderly way, the process is rarely tidy; action researchers might find themselves rethinking, repeating, or revising steps in the process (Ladkin, 2007; Stringer, 2007). The action research spiral represents a dialectical relationship between retrospective understanding

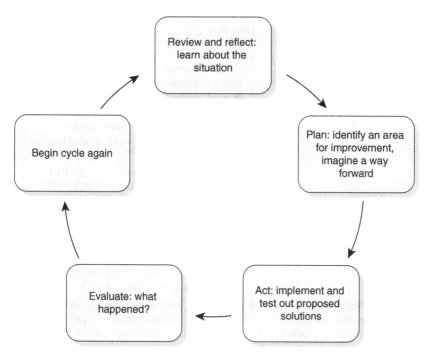

Figure 8.1 A typical cycle of action research

and prospective action (Carr & Kemmis, 1986). Thus action researchers at each moment "look back" as a basis for reflection and "look forward" for realization of the plan in action (Carr & Kemmis, 1986). Two action–reflection cycles is generally considered the minimum level of engagement necessary for useful and meaningful change to occur (Kemmis & McTaggart, 1988).

Topics and questions suited to action research

Practice and practice knowledge are multifaceted concepts that are not easily studied using traditional scientific methods (Schön, 1995) but explorations of practices and practice settings are well suited to examination using action research (Kemmis, 2005; Shotter, 2000). As practices are complex, the research questions that are explored through action research may also be comprehensive and multifaceted; who, what, why, where, and how, are often included in action research questions (refer Table 8.1).

Recruitment and sampling

Action research is collaborative; therefore, the issue of recruitment and sampling in action research is influenced by the role that each person takes. In classic forms

Table 8.1 Examples of action research topics and questions

Topic	Questions
1 Exploring issues of power and oppression, occupational justice, community development, and supporting marginalized peoples	a How do occupational therapists understand and enact human rights and occupational justice in a hospital context? What contextual features constrain the practice of enabling rights and justice, and how might these be transformed into other, desired conditions, and practices? (Galvin, Wilding, & Whiteford, 2011, p. 379)
	b What insights can be gained, into the barriers inhibiting the effectiveness of a support and self-help group for women who are carers of children with disabilities? (Adams & Galvaan, 2010, p. 13)
	c How can an occupational therapy program be developed to facilitate school participation with adolescents from refugee backgrounds? (Copley, Turpin, Gordon, & McLaren, 2011, p. 310)
2 Exploring how occupational theory and evidence can be applied in occupational therapy practice	a How is the Canadian Model of Occupational Performance implemented in occupational therapy practice? (Boniface et al., 2008, p. 352)
	b How can barriers to theory integration be removed? . . . What is the impact of the Model of Human Occupation upon therapists' perception of their role and on their practice? (Wimpenny, Forsyth, Jones, Evans, & Colley, 2010, p. 508)
3 Exploring entrenched practice problems and exposing taken-for-granted aspects of practice	a How can the impacts of theory utilization, evidence utilization, and occupation-focus be better understood in relation to articulation of occupational therapy? And therefore, what is the experience of the use of theory, use of evidence, and use of occupation as perceived by a group of occupational therapists working in an acute practice setting, and how do the occupational therapists make sense of these issues in their everyday practices? (Wilding, 2008, p. 51)

of participatory action research, all people who are participating in the action research process are also researchers (or co-researchers); a group of people *decide* together to research their shared life-world. Thus, rather than recruiting a sample of participants, a group of researchers *form together* to examine the shared situation that is the topic of interest in the action research.

There are forms of action research that, while being collaborative, also allow for different members of the research group to take on different roles. Danika took on a research leadership role and recruited co-researchers who were occupational therapists from a hospital where Danika had not previously worked. Danika is an occupational therapist with 12 years of experience working in medical practice settings, particularly in rehabilitation with people who have an acquired brain injury. The research group formed to investigate their shared values about iniquitous occupational issues and absences of occupational rights in occupational therapy practice. All researchers were interested in exploring how the occupational science concept, occupational justice, could be applied to improve their practice. The self-selected co-researchers agreed to become engaged in cycles of action research; they consented to reflect on their practice, discuss their practice with others, and plan and take actions of their choosing. Danika's role differed from those of the others, in that as part of her doctoral studies, she took responsibility for coordinating research meetings, collecting and analyzing data, and ultimately reporting her findings as a thesis.

If one or more researchers take a research leadership role, it is important to realize that the power differential can affect the collaboration and therefore care needs to be taken so that one person's perspective does not dominate or impose unduly on the perspectives of others. Freire (1970) stressed that if a person in a position of power attempted to tell others how to act, no transformation would occur, because in order to enact real change, a person needed to develop self-awareness of the situation and through this deepened understanding of the situation would be inspired to act. The aim of action research is not to change others but for each person to take responsibility for making changes to his or her own situation (McNiff & Whitehead, 2010). Thus "social change happens when people think for themselves and mobilise themselves for action" (McNiff, 2013, p. 10).

Data collection

Within action research, qualitative and/or quantitative data may be collected. Thus, methods of data collection are varied and may include interviews, focus groups, surveys, population statistics, participant observation, or collection of other forms of texts or practice artifacts. Action research is an ongoing process of reflection, discovery, testing out new discoveries, and re-evaluation; therefore, data collection and data analysis occur simultaneously. However, Kemmis and McTaggart (1988) advocated that action research ought to be undertaken in a systematic and reflective way, in order that important steps in the process are not overlooked. The four steps in the action research cycle and the data collection that occurred at each stage of the process will be profiled as it related to Danika's study (Table 8.2).

Step 1: review and reflect

Danika interviewed each of the eight occupational therapists who agreed to explore with her how human rights and occupational justice influenced

Table 8.2 Cycles of data collection in Danika's action research study

Action research step	Data collected
1 Review and reflect	Transcripts of interviews
	Transcripts of focus groups
2 Plan	Transcripts of focus groups
3 Act	Transcripts of interviews
	Transcripts of focus groups
4 Evaluate	Transcripts of interviews
	Transcripts of focus groups

their practice. The focus of these interviews was to prompt reflection about the therapists' previous practice background and their needs and desires for learning and change. Following completion of the interviews, Danika established a shared communicative space by forming a focus group of all participating therapists. This research group met monthly for between 60 and 90 minutes (for a total of 10 months). During the first four groups, the action researchers considered what human rights and occupational justice were (Textbox 8.1) and how they were relevant to their practice. The interviews and the group discussions were audio-recorded and the transcribed texts were collected as data.

Textbox 8.1 Sample focus group questions: review and reflect

- What is your vision of ideal occupational therapy practice?
- What significance do human rights and occupational justice have in this vision?
- How does this vision fit with the reality of your practice?
- What responsibility do you have to enact rights and justice in practice?
- What is the potential to change your practice in order to positively promote rights and justice?

Step 2: plan

The second step of the action research spiral pertains to planning "where to act to produce the most powerful effect compatible with sustaining the struggle of reform" (Kemmis & McTaggart, 1988, p. 65) and is about developing a strong understanding of a plan and signaling an intention and commitment to act. In Danika's study, the research group considered what was to be done about their practice situation, including about what, by whom, where, when, and how. Focus groups five to seven were dedicated to planning for change (Textbox 8.2).

Textbox 8.2   Sample focus group questions: plan

- What kinds of human rights issues evoke your interest?
- How will you make a difference through enabling occupation and justice?
- What changes will you need to make to your own knowledge?
- What changes will you make to the systems and processes in which you work?
- What supports (e.g., mentors, literature) will help you to achieve your vision?
- Will you take this action individually or with others inside/outside the group?
- How will you monitor your actions and the effect it has?

Step 3: act

In the third step, action researchers need to simultaneously adhere to enacting their plan and remain open to modifying the plan so that it better meets the immediate circumstances and conditions of the change (Kemmis & McTaggart, 1988). It is important to closely observe what is happening as a basis for ongoing reflection. Danika facilitated the reflections of the action researchers by engaging them in individual and group discussions about their experiences of implementing actions to enhance occupational justice.

Step 4: evaluate

The final step of the action research spiral is to evaluate the effects of the action that has been taken. In this step, the action researchers reflected upon whether the actions they had taken were relevant to, and appropriate for, enabling occupational justice in their practice. In a final set of individual interviews and focus group meetings, the action researchers considered which conditions enabled or constrained occupationally just practice and discussed what they had learned and what else they needed to learn (Textbox 8.3).

Textbox 8.3   Sample focus group questions: act and evaluate

- What changes have you made to your practice over the past month?
- What has worked well and what could have been done differently?
- What effect did this have (either positive or negative) on you or upon others around you?
- For those who have not yet started to enact your plan, why has this been difficult to do and what supports do you require?
- What do you plan to do next? Will you continue on, stop to revise your action plan and try again, or do something else?

Although the research group as a whole moved through two cycles of action research, the implementation of the cycles was not so neatly formed or consistent for individual researchers. In the final 3 months of the study, some researchers completed multiple shorter length (one month-long) cycles, whereas others struggled to engage completely in two cycles because they experienced challenges in identifying where to start making their desired changes.

Data analysis

Data analysis in action research can be a complex process as there may be multiple data sources, and data may not be analyzed in a linear way but rather as layers of data analysis that occur simultaneously. In addition, there may be more than one researcher analyzing the data and different researchers may be working with different data sets and be at different stages and levels of analysis at any particular point in time. Thus, data analysis may include a group of co-researchers' private, public, individual, and collective analyses, which may also be shared and reflected upon (individually and collectively) as the action research spiral proceeds.

As action research is a process of learning, using the learning to inform action, and reflecting on the action taken to stimulate further learning, it is best if data analysis begins almost immediately. Once started, data analysis will continue throughout the study. Data analysis will yield changes in the researchers' understandings and this new knowledge is used to inform action planning and implementation (and further data collection). Findings ought to be discussed and critiqued as they emerge throughout the life of the action research study. Through this process of sharing and developing findings concurrently with generating and collecting data, it may be seen that the analyses become folded back in on themselves.

Data analysis may consist of both formal, systematic, and structured analysis and informal, less structured analysis. Formal analysis uses any recognized data analysis method that the researcher chooses; for example, a hermeneutic phenomenological or grounded theory or discourse analysis. Informal analysis is a less structured creative activity in which the researcher spends time thinking about, pondering, and developing understanding of the research situation. These processes are not really separate, as one informs the other; however, it is important to realize that just as action research is complex, so too is the data analysis process. Formal and informal analysis processes can be used to achieve "a mix of creativity and order" (Marshall, 2002, p. 68).

Clare's (Wilding, 2008) study illustrates use of formal and informal analysis processes. Clare is an experienced occupational therapist. She provided occupational therapy services for people who had mental illness during the first 7 years of her occupational therapy career. Then, she worked for more than 16 years as an Australian academic, with a mix of roles teaching occupational therapy, in academic leadership, and as a researcher. During her doctoral studies, Clare engaged with a group of 15 occupational therapists in an action research of occupational therapy practice in an Australian metropolitan hospital. Clare collected narrative data through individual interviews and group discussions.

Data were formally analyzed using line-by-line coding and thematic analysis. First, the transcripts were read and re-read and hand-written codes were created in the margins. The codes commenced with a verb that described the main action, feeling, or thought and used language that was the same or very similar to that used by the speaker of the selected passage. Next, Clare clustered and chunked the codes, assigning each cluster a new category title. Initially, using lists of categories and codes and the word-processing software, *Microsoft Word*, and later using mind-mapping software, *Free Mind*, Clare compared and contrasted, sorted, and organized and re-organized the categories and codes from each transcript into a mosaic that partially described and explained the occupational therapy practice that was the focus of the research.

Clare also conducted informal analysis using her research diary, case stories provided by the co-researchers, preliminary findings documents, and a monthly news sheet about the research; this analysis involved reading and re-reading these artifacts, making notes about them, using them to generate more research questions, and discussing the artifacts with the co-researchers and her supervisors. The dual processes of formal and informal analysis enabled deep reflection upon the research issues and were used as a stimulus for discussion in research group meetings.

Similar to the process of data analysis, presenting the findings of action research is often complex and multilayered and may require a mix of systematic and creative approaches. Findings ought to be presented in the style that is most appropriate to the methods that were used to analyze the data (e.g., phenomenology, grounded theory, discourse analysis). However, when presenting the findings about what was learned about the particular problems or issues that were the focus of the study, researchers may also like to include an overall account of the learning journey they went through during the course of the study. A metaphor may be useful to help illustrate complex ideas in a concise way. For example, Clare conceptualized the overall journey portrayed in her study as one of moving from initial enchantment with occupation-focused occupational therapy practice through dis-enchantment and ultimately to re-enchantment. Danika theorized that the process of creating occupational justice involved first finding out about where the path to occupational justice ought to be and what it looked like, then making a commitment to build the path, and lastly, walking the new path.

Ethics

The ethical issues relevant to conducting action research include ensuring the study adheres to recognized research processes and seeking independent review of the proposed processes; ensuring the study has scientific or social value; choosing co-researchers who will gain the most benefit from involvement; balancing risks and benefits; obtaining informed consent; and, demonstrating respect for those who participate in the study (Khanlou & Peter, 2005). In action research, considering these ethical issues may be complicated by the collaborative relationships and unfolding nature that constitutes this type of research. Given that action research is a broad approach to research rather than a prescribed set of activities, the onus lies with the researchers responsible for each individual study to clearly describe and justify the proposed specific methods that will be used.

As previously mentioned, there can be considerable variation regarding the ways in which the collaborative relationships and the different roles of the researchers are constituted. Hence, sometimes the methods that will be used have been mapped out in advance and sometimes these methods are determined during the course of the study. In our studies, because we were both student researchers, we had already decided the shape and length of our studies from the outset of the research and therefore we were able to clearly describe in our ethics applications how the research would be conducted, how co-researchers would be recruited and respected, and the risk–benefit ratio for the research and co-researchers. Providing a clear overview of how the research would proceed facilitated gaining ethical approval. In studies that invite co-researchers to help shape the way in which information is collected and therefore the research methods may not be known in advance, ethics approval may need to be sought for each cycle of the research process (Khanlou & Peter, 2005).

Action research is situated research; thus much of the value of the research can lie in the context-embedded understandings that are developed. However, such specificity can make confidentiality and anonymity difficult to achieve. This might not be problematic if a group of authors take responsibility for reporting the study's findings, since then they can choose how to portray themselves in their reporting, including what will be reported and what is kept confidential. In studies like ours, we had an obligation to produce theses as research outcomes, which needed to be our own original work and therefore anonymity and confidentiality were addressed by seeking informed consent and taking steps to help mask co-researchers' identities. Informed consent was addressed through providing clear information sheets about the research, which detailed the requirements of participation. In addition, we conducted briefing meetings for potential co-researchers to describe and discuss the research. In the theses and reporting of the studies, pseudonyms were used to help mask the co-researchers' identities, and we took care to avoid inadvertently exposing any particular person's identity.

Rigor

High-quality action research does not come from slavish adherence to a particular technique, as there is considerable flexibility available within this approach to research. Rather, it is the attitude and orientation that a researcher brings with him or her that must be closely held to. It is not "the machinery of research techniques" that makes action research "research" (Kemmis & McTaggart, 2000, p. 33) but rather a culture of critical inquiry (Mattson & Kemmis, 2007). Thus, it is vital that researchers keep to the fore the philosophical ideals and essential qualities of action research: those of critical self-reflection, collaboration, dialog, emancipation and transformation, learning, and social justice.

Action research ought to stimulate critical reflection (Mattson & Kemmis, 2007). Danika facilitated critical thinking by providing reflection questions that encouraged co-researchers to think deeply about their own perspectives prior to joining with the other researchers in the monthly group discussions. She also encouraged co-researchers to share and discuss their practice stories during the research group discussions; Osler and Zhu (2011) asserted that telling previously untold stories may enable practitioners to more closely understand others' human experience and practice, which can prompt reflections upon their own values and beliefs in relation to justice.

Strategies commonly used for ensuring trustworthiness in qualitative research that are relevant to action research include triangulation, reflexivity, peer review, supervision, and keeping an audit trail. Triangulation through utilizing a range of different data sources and/or methods may be used. For example, a mix of qualitative methods (such as case story *and* thematic analysis) may be used and/or quantitative methods (such as surveys or outcome measurement tools or specific assessment tools) may be *added* to qualitative methods of data collection and analysis.

Liamputtong and Ezzy (2005) asserted that writing in a reflective diary (or field journal) is a common and useful means of promoting reflexivity. A reflective diary might include a record of emerging ideas about the research; responses to literature reviewed; pre-understandings and developing understandings of the research issues; questions and ideas to consider; reflections on interviews; and reflections on field visits. Meeting regularly with supervisors, or critical colleagues, or a reference group for peer debriefing can further develop reflexivity. Presenting preliminary findings that are critiqued by others can also facilitate reflexivity, as this process forces a researcher to think about what is happening in the research and to form his or her thoughts into a coherent format that is understandable to others.

Use of an audit trail enables transparency and replication of a study. As action research is a complex process, it is likely that an audit trail will consist of a suite of documents, rather than a singular source. For example, Clare (Wilding, 2008) included the following documents in her audit trail portfolio: a reflective diary; an appointment diary; minutes of meetings with supervisors; notes of meetings with co-researchers; a record of communications with co-researchers; preliminary findings documents; and monthly news sheets about the research that were shared with co-researchers.

Critiquing action research studies

When critiquing studies that purport to have used action research, a reader should take note of who the researchers are and how research roles have been distributed in the research team. There ought to be naming of the specific methods of data collection and analysis. The actions that were taken to achieve critical and emancipatory change should also be clearly described. Questions that can be used to critique action research studies appear in Textbox 8.4.

Textbox 8.4 Critiquing action research studies – questions to ask

1 Have the *researchers' positions* been made explicit? Who is in the research team? What roles have different members of the team taken?
2 *Whose analysis* is being presented?
3 How has *power been shared* by the researchers?
4 Which *particular methods* have been selected? Are the methods of data collection and data analysis sufficiently described?
5 *How many cycles of action research* were implemented? (Are there at least two cycles)?
6 What has been learned and how has this knowledge been used to *transform the life-worlds* of the participants? (What has been discovered and what actions have these discoveries inspired?)
7 What techniques have been used to promote researchers to be critical, reflective, and collaborative? How has *communication and dialog* between researchers been facilitated?

Application to occupational science

Action research is an excellent means by which to explore complex and situated phenomena and practices, such as occupational science and occupational therapy. The action research process of discovery, trialing action to make change, and then examining the effects of this change makes it a methodology that is well suited to exploring everyday situations and experiences without stripping away the context that so vitally informs everyday life. Therefore, action research provides an effective way of exploring occupations and testing out emergent occupational science concepts. Danika's study applied action research in this way (Textbox 8.5).

Textbox 8.5 Action research in occupational science

A study that explored the concept of occupational justice and how occupational therapists apply this construct in their practice (in part reported in Galvin et al., 2011)

Danika's research enabled action researchers to engage in local, contextualized dialog about the conditions and practices that hinder human rights and occupational justice. Through this process of learning and critique, action researchers were able to act to transform these practice conditions in accordance with their desire to enable occupational justice.

Not only did the implementation of occupational science concepts contribute to new practices for occupational justice, the action researchers constructed new, localized, contextualized meanings about occupational justice, thus demonstrating the potential of a discursive approach to further shaping occupational science knowledge.

Application to occupational therapy

Action research is ideally suited to examine and change many types of practice, including occupational therapy. When engaging in action research about practice, practitioners become action researchers and their practice becomes the situation that is being investigated. It is a form of inquiry that can enable practitioners to work through the complex issues and problems that they face and make their work more meaningful and fulfilling (Stringer, 2007). When used by practitioners, action research has the potential to be a tool that enables improved practice and emancipation through enlightenment of practice arrangements (Kemmis, 2006). By critiquing and learning about the conditions that produce particular practices and that are reproduced in everyday social interaction, practitioners become alert to clues about how to make and re-make other, more desired circumstances and practices (Kemmis & McTaggart, 2005). Clare's study applied action research in this way (Textbox 8.6).

Textbox 8.6   Action research in occupational therapy

A study of how occupational therapists explain occupational therapy and use occupation in their practice in a hospital setting (Wilding, 2008).

Clare's research problematized taken-for-granted ways in which occupational therapists thought about, talked about, and enacted their occupational therapy practice. Through this process of learning and critique, the action researchers were able to transform their thinking, talking, and doing such that their practice was more occupation-focused.

The value of action research in this case was that it assisted the occupational therapists to recognize their unconscious hegemony and through making their realization they were able to more consciously craft the kind of practice that fitted better with their philosophies and values.

Cockburn and Trentham (2002) pointed to a closeness of fit between action research and occupational therapy, citing values such as being client-centered, working collaboratively, and facilitating learning through action as ones that action research and occupational therapy hold in common.

Reflections on using action research

We found using action research to be a very complex and flexible process and this meant that engaging in action research was simultaneously challenging, exciting, and extremely useful. Managing a complex process takes time and effort. We discovered that it was important to be organized. It was also best to be well-prepared *and* be willing to discard one's plan when circumstances changed, which was invariably the case. Although such unpredictability was unsettling, we realized that in such a fluid environment it was easy to get interested in what was happening and seek to understand why, how, and what created the situations that were experienced. Being interested in the research made it easy to stay focused, engaged, and committed and to seek out the answers to the research questions.

We also valued the highly practical and contextualized nature of action research. It is learning that is bespoke and therefore we found that it produced highly relevant answers to the thorny occupational science and occupational therapy practice questions that we were seeking answers for. It is not only theoretical understanding that is gained, knowledge of *how* to create change is a valuable by-product of action research. In addition, for the researchers there was no delay for knowledge translation; the process of engaging in the research included discovering, understanding, contextualizing, and using the knowledge that was learned and applying it immediately to the practice situation.

We appreciated the benefits that were gained through the collaborative nature of action research. Through this teamwork, we were able to fuse academic and practice goals and agendas. Each person in the cooperative was able to bring his or her own different and important perspective to bear upon the problematic issue that was being studied, and we consider that this strengthened the research findings. The practitioner–academic alliances that we established during our action research studies fitted well with our personal values and thus we experienced engaging in action research to be highly satisfying.

Challenges to using action research

Action research is sometimes criticized for creating unsustainable change; after the process is completed it may be difficult for researchers to maintain their commitment to and implementation of the actions that they created while the study was being undertaken. Maintaining a commitment to change in a hostile environment without a support group is certainly very difficult. In our experience, it can be very challenging to maintain occupation-focused and occupationally just practice in health services in which the medical model is the dominant ideology. In addition, some occupational therapists may find hegemonic discourses hard to resist (Wilding, 2011). Thus, philosophical mismatch and conflict are significant challenges and can create an ongoing struggle for sustaining transformation that has been initiated during an action research.

Although creating sustainable change can be complex, we consider that there are strategies that can be used to increase the likelihood that change is maintained over time. It can be useful to implement an action research over a prolonged period of time (e.g., 12–18 months). A lengthy period of action research means that participating therapists will have invested significantly in reflection, discussion, and building relationships with their co-researchers. There will have been plenty of time to understand the practice situation and its problems, time for supported efforts at change, and time for addressing a range of practice problems. Change is more likely to be sustained if there has been a critical mass of therapists in the department or service who participated in the action research. Also, if the action research included senior members/leaders of the occupational therapy department/service, sustained change may be more likely because this mass of therapists and leaders may create cultural change. A third strategy for sustaining change is to create practice artifacts and resources for practice that support the transformed practice. For example, creating a webpage that describes the occupational therapy service in an occupation-focused way or changing an assessment tool to include an assessment of occupational justice issues.

Conclusion: the rewards of action research

Action research is a powerful way of learning, taking action, and ultimately transforming practice. It can be a very creative and liberating process and in the long term this is deeply satisfying. Action research is a contextually relevant form of research that may be specifically tailored to a particular organization or group's practice. The specialized learning achieved through this type of purpose-built research can have deep meaning and significance for the research settings in which action research is undertaken.

Action research is research that is social; engaging with other action researchers can be very inspiring and motivating. Creativity may be sparked through dialog and discussion. A group of researchers working in collaboration may develop a greater level of insight and achieve more than is possible for a solitary researcher. A sense of collegiality and camaraderie can make dealing with difficult and problematic situations easier and less stressful. Indeed, it may be said that it is possible to have fun completing action research, even as more serious aims of deepening knowledge and creating practice change are achieved.

References

Adams, F., & Galvaan, R. (2010). Promoting human rights: Understanding the barriers to self-help groups for women who are carers of children with disabilities. *South African Journal of Occupational Therapy, 40*(1), 12–16.

Boniface, G., Fedden, T., Hurst, H., Mason, M., Phelps, C., Reagon, C., & Waygood, S. (2008). Using theory to underpin an integrated occupational therapy service through the Canadian Model of Occupational Performance. *British Journal of Occupational Therapy, 71*(12), 531–539.

Bray, J. N., Lee, J., Smith, L. L., & Yorks, L. (2000). *Collaborative inquiry in practice.* Thousand Oaks, CA: Sage.

Carr, W. (2009). Practice without theory? A postmodern perspective on educational practice. In B. Green (Ed.), *Understanding and researching professional practice* (pp. 55–64). Rotterdam, Netherlands: Sense Publishers.

Carr, W., & Kemmis, S. (1986). *Becoming critical: Education, knowledge and action research.* London, UK: Routledge Falmer.

Cockburn, L., & Trentham, B. (2002). Participatory action research: Integrating community occupational therapy practice and research. *Canadian Journal of Occupational Therapy, 69*, 20–30.

Copley, J., Turpin, M., Gordon, S., & McLaren, C. (2011). Development and evaluation of an occupational therapy program for refugee high school students. *Australian Occupational Therapy Journal, 58*, 310–316. doi:10.1111/j.1440-1630.2011.00933.x.

Freire, P. (1970). *Pedagogy of the oppressed.* New York, NY: Seabury Press.

Galvin, D., Wilding, C., & Whiteford, G. (2011). Utopian visions/dystopian realities: Exploring practice and taking action to enable human rights and occupational justice in a hospital context. *Australian Occupational Therapy Journal, 58*(5), 378–385. doi:10.1111/j.1440-1630.2011.00967.x.

Gaventa, J., & Cornwall, A. (2006). Power and knowledge. In P. Reason & H. Bradbury (Eds.), *Handbook of action research: Concise paperback edition* (pp. 71–82). Los Angeles, CA: Sage.

Gustavsen, B. (2006). Theory and practice: The mediating discourse. In P. Reason & H. Bradbury (Eds.), *Handbook of action research: Concise paperback edition* (pp. 17–26). Los Angeles, CA: Sage.

Ife, J. (2008). *Human rights and social work: Towards rights-based practice* (2nd ed.). Cambridge, UK: Cambridge University Press.

Kemmis, S. (2005). Knowing practice: Searching for saliences. *Pedagogy, Culture and Society, 13*(3), 391–426.

Kemmis, S. (2006). Exploring the relevance of critical theory for action research: Emancipatory action research in the footsteps of Jurgen Habermas. In P. Reason, & H. Bradbury (Eds.), *Handbook of action research: Participative inquiry and practice* (pp. 91–102). London, UK: Sage.

Kemmis, S., & McTaggart, R. (1988). *The action research planner* (3rd Rev. ed.). Waurn Ponds, Australia: Deakin University.

Kemmis, S., & McTaggart, R. (2000). Participatory action research. In N. Denzin & Y. Lincoln (Eds.), *The Sage handbook of qualitative research* (2nd ed., pp. 567–605). Beverly Hills, CA: Sage.

Kemmis, S., & McTaggart, R. (2005). Participatory action research: Communicative action and the public sphere. In N. Denzin & Y. Lincoln (Eds.), *The Sage handbook of qualitative research* (3rd ed., pp. 559–603). Thousand Oaks, CA: Sage.

Khanlou, N., & Peter, E. (2005). Participatory action research: Considerations for ethical review. *Social Science and Medicine, 60*, 2333–2340. doi:10.1016/j.socscimed. 2004.10.004.

Klein, S. R. (Ed.). (2012). *Action research methods: Plain and simple.* New York, NY: Palgrave Macmillan.

Koch, T., & Kralik, D. (2001). Chronic illness: Reflections on a community-based action research programme. *Journal of Advanced Nursing, 36*, 23–31. doi:10.1046/j.1365-2648. 2001.01939.x.

Koch, T., Selim, P., & Kralik, D. (2002). Enhancing lives through the development of a community-based participatory action research programme. *Journal of Clinical Nursing, 11*, 109–117. doi:10.1046/j.1365-2702.2002.00563.x.

Ladkin, D. (2007). Action research. In C. Seale, G. Gobo, J. Gubrium, & D. Silverman (Eds.), *Qualitative research practice* (pp. 478–490). London, UK: Sage.

Liamputtong, P., & Ezzy, D. (2005). *Qualitative research methods* (2nd ed.). Oxford, UK: Oxford University Press.

Ludema, J., Cooperrider, D., & Barrett, F. (2006). Appreciative inquiry: The power of the unconditional positive question. In P. Reason & H. Bradbury (Eds.), *Handbook of action research: Concise paperback edition* (pp. 155–165). Los Angeles, CA: Sage.

Marshall, H. (2002). What do we do when we code data? *Qualitative Research Journal, 2*(1), 56–70.

Mattson, M., & Kemmis, S. (2007). Praxis-related research: Serving two masters? *Pedagogy, Culture & Society, 15*(2), 185–214. doi:10.1080/14681360701403706.

McNiff, J. (2013). *Action research: Principles and practice* (3rd ed.). London, UK: Routledge.

McNiff, J., & Whitehead, J. (2010). *You and your action research project* (3rd ed.). London, UK: Routledge.

Osler, A., & Zhu, J. (2011). Narratives in teaching and research for justice and human rights. *Education, Citizenship and Social Justice, 6*, 223–235. doi:10.1177/1746197911417414.

Reason, P., & Bradbury, H. (2006). Introduction: Inquiry and participation in search of a world worthy of human aspiration. In P. Reason & H. Bradbury (Eds.), *Handbook of action research: Concise paperback edition* (pp. 1–14). Los Angeles, CA: Sage.

Schön, D. A. (1995). The new scholarship requires a new epistemology. *Change, 27*(6), 26–34.

Shotter, J. (2000). From within our lives together: Wittgenstein, Bakhtin, and Voloshinov and the shift to a participatory stance in understanding understanding. In L. Holzman & J. Morss (Eds.), *Postmodern psychologies, societal practice, and political life* (pp. 100–129). New York, NY: Routledge.

Soltis-Jarrett, V. (1997). The facilitator in participatory action research: Les raisons d'être. *Advances in Nursing Science, 20*(2), 45–54.

Stringer, E. (2007). *Action research* (3rd ed.). Los Angeles, CA: Sage.

Townsend, E., Birch, D. E., Langley, J., & Langille, L. (2000). Participatory research in a mental health clubhouse. *Occupational Therapy Journal of Research, 20*, 18–44.

Wilding, C. (2008). *Identifying, articulating, and transforming occupational therapy practice in an acute setting: A collaborative action research study.* Unpublished doctoral thesis, Charles Sturt University, Albury, NSW, Australia.

Wilding, C. (2011). Raising awareness of hegemony in occupational therapy: The value of action research for improving practice. *Australian Occupational Therapy Journal, 58*(4), 293–299.

Wimpenny, K., Forsyth, K., Jones, C., Matheson, L., & Colley, J. (2010). Implementing the Model of Human Occupation across a mental health occupational therapy service: Communities of practice and a participatory change process. *British Journal of Occupational Therapy, 73*(11), 507–516. doi:http://dx.doi.org/10.4276/030802210X12892992239152.

Further reading

Action Research Journal: arj.sagepub.com/

Bryant, W., McKay, E., Beresford, P., & Vacher, G. (2011). An occupational perspective on participatory action research. In F. Kronenberg, N. Pollard, & D. Sakellariou (Eds.), *Occupational therapies without borders: Towards an ecology of occupation-based practices* (Vol. 2, pp. 368–374). Edinburgh, Scotland: Churchill Livingstone Elsevier.

Reed, K., & Hocking, C. (2013). Re-visioning practice through action research. *Australian Occupational Therapy Journal, 60*, 181–188. doi:10.1111/1440–1630.12033.

Websites

Collaborative Action Research Network (CARN): http://www.esri.mmu.ac.uk/carnnew/index.php

Jean McNiff's website: http://www.jeanmcniff.com/

9 Case study methodology
The particular and the whole

Margaret Jones and Clare Hocking

Textbox 9.1   Tish

Rugby, a ball game played in teams, is central to the Northwood rural community. Tish was a skilled player in the school team, until he was hit by a car on his way to practice 2 years ago. Now he isn't allowed to play, and school work is hard for him too. The other team members are going away for a week on a rugby trip. Tish isn't allowed to go. When Margaret asked him about it, he said rugby is dumb, and he didn't want to go anyway. His father hopes Tish will be allowed to play next year.

Occupational scientists and therapists are concerned with the ways people like Tish (Textbox 9.1) engage in unique patterns of occupation that are interwoven with the fabric of their communities. Case study methodology provides a means of exploring the particulars of these occupations, at the same time as they are bound together as a whole within the contexts in which people go about their everyday lives. In writing this chapter, we share our experiences of case study methodology. We explain the ways the methodology was applied when we studied children's participation in occupations after they sustain a brain injury.

Background

The term *case study* is often thought to have begun with the use of social workers' case notes in early social science research. Over time the term has been used to denote fieldwork, observations, case reports, ethnography, and illustrative case examples developed for teaching. Some have believed case studies are merely precursors to more comprehensive research projects (Platt, 1992), while others have argued that case study is not a research method but is more a choice about *what* will be studied (Hesse-Biber & Leavy, 2011).

Concurring with Cresswell (2007), we will refer to case study as a methodology. As illustrated in Figure 9.1, although case studies do focus inquiry on a case or cases, they also share a common intent, specific strategies and processes, and

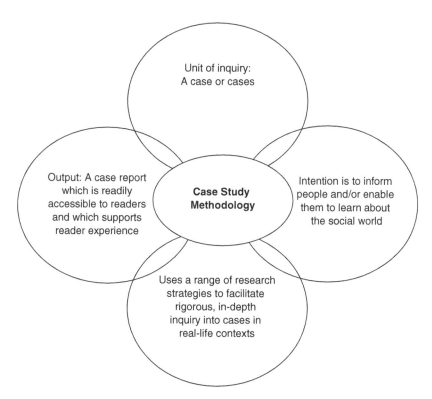

Figure 9.1 Case study methodology

careful consideration of the audience when generating outputs (Cresswell, 2007; Merriam, 2009; Simons, 2009; Stake, 1995; Yin, 2009).

Case study methodology is diversely applied in fields such as sociology, anthropology, psychology, education, nursing, political science, law, business, policy (Hammersly & Gomm, 2000; Platt, 1992; Yin, 2009), and occupational science and therapy (Cameron et al., 2013; Smith, Stephenson, & Gibson-Satterthwaite, 2013). The different applications of case study research complicate its definition. However, Yin (2009) usefully defined case study as an "empirical inquiry" which "investigates a contemporary phenomenon in depth and within its real-life context" particularly where "the boundaries between phenomenon and context are not clearly evident" (p. 18).

A case or cases are the focus of the investigation. The "case" in case study is a natural, functioning, material phenomenon. It is situated in a particular context and time, a thing that can be experienced. The case may center on an individual person, a group or community, an organization or political entity, or multiple groups that share a common feature such as experience of a certain event. Because cases are intertwined with their contexts, even a single person case is regarded as a system (Stake, 1995; Yin, 2009).

Case study research is concerned with addressing people's practical day-to-day doings and their experiences of those doings, rather than abstracts or metaphysical notions. The concern with the real-life doings of humans in context suggests the methodology is well suited for increasing knowledge about people's occupations. Occupational scientists and therapists who have a transactional perspective (Cutchin & Dickie, 2013) will relate to the way a case study can tease out and make sense of the multiple and complex interactions between people and their environments.

There are numerous instances of case studies in the literature, although closer examination shows that most of these are case reports or illustrations, rather than formal research projects. Nonetheless, examples of recent reports of case study methodology include the following: in occupational science, examining traditional weaving occupations (Smith et al., 2013); and in occupational therapy, primary care (Donnelly, Brenchley, Crawford, & Letts, 2013), international partnerships in postgraduate programs (Ilott et al., 2013), patient handling (Darragh et al., 2013), and fieldwork innovations (Cameron et al., 2013; Provident & Comer, 2013).

Approaching the research topic

Our concern with children's participation after traumatic brain injury (TBI) arose from Margaret's occupational therapy practice in a pediatric rehabilitation setting. Both authors were aware that despite rehabilitation to enhance children's occupational performance, they continued to have difficulty taking part in occupations when they returned to their communities. We believed that participation was important but did not know whether the families shared our beliefs. We were unsure what contributed to the children's participation difficulties, let alone knowing the most appropriate way to address them.

A review of the rehabilitation literature generated few answers. Although some research had been conducted internationally, it showed variability in the way participation outcomes were conceptualized. There were also variable outcomes across different settings, suggesting that findings generated in other geographical and cultural contexts may not apply to children in New Zealand. Most studies involved parent perspectives, and only a limited number explored data from the children, teachers, or support staff. Few interventions were documented that directly addressed participation.

Case study methodology seemed to mesh with our practical need to learn in greater detail about children's participation in the New Zealand setting. It aligned with our view of participation as connected with both occupation and context and with the need to gather information from more than one person's perspective.

Types of case study

Different types of case studies elicit design variations according to their purpose. There are exploratory, descriptive, explanatory, or evaluative case studies (Merriam, 2009; Stake, 1995, 2006; Yin, 2009). As illustrated in Figure 9.2, Stake

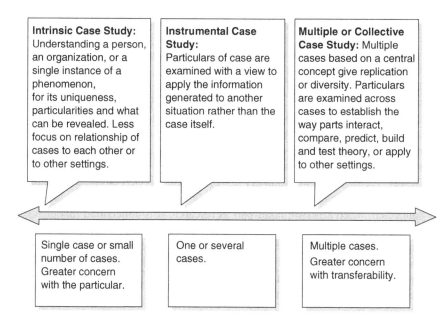

Figure 9.2 Continuum of case study designs. Developed from Stake (1995, 2006)

(1995, 2006) further proposed that case studies can be considered as intrinsic, instrumental, or multiple. The process of identifying the best type of case study to use for our own research provoked much deliberation. Our decision was aided by the theoretical perspectives that informed the project.

Epistemology

Consistent with the diverse uses of case study methodology, there is no one underlying theoretical perspective. Some case studies reflect a positivist perspective, often with intent to test theory or to explain cause and effect relationships (Gerring, 2007; Yin, 2009). Such studies fall outside the scope of this chapter. Case studies may adopt a critical position, exposing oppression and driving social change. Other case studies may adopt an interpretivist perspective, such as ethnographic projects concerned with understanding a cultural group (Merriam, 2009).

Whatever the theoretical perspective, it will shape the research questions, the number of cases, the data sources used, the type of information sought, and the approach to data analysis. Explicating the theoretical perspective that informs the case study enables others to see the position the researcher adopted toward the project and to appreciate the reasons behind decisions made at various points in the research process.

The theoretical perspective that guided our own case study research was the pragmatist philosophy of John Dewey. This philosophy is concerned with practical and moral outcomes of human knowledge. Dewey believed that people learn through doing things in response to problems encountered as part of a changing world. Although he recognized that human experiences have unique meanings for different individuals, he also acknowledged the importance of sharing experiences with others (Dewey, 1916, 1925/1981).

This perspective informed our goal of understanding people's experiences of children's participation after TBI and the things which were of practical assistance. We hoped to generate strategies to support the children's participation and broaden others' knowledge. Although we acknowledged that each case would be unique, the focus was application of the information to other situations; therefore an instrumental case study was proposed.

Dewey's pragmatist philosophy (1925/1981) also directed our understandings about our roles as researchers. Because people and their environments are seen as connected, when a person takes part in research, it is understood that change occurs in both the person and the environment. Therefore, when Margaret was gathering data, rather than setting herself apart, she interacted as seemed natural, acknowledging in her written reflections the ways in which she influenced the information generated. Data were therefore viewed as being co-constructed between the researcher and participants.

Developing the research questions

Within case study methodology, research questions (sometimes referred to as issue questions) perform an important role in organizing the study. Yin (2009) explained that case studies are well suited for answering "how" or "why" questions but that they are also useful to answer "what" questions where the study is exploratory in nature.

In some situations, a researcher may be requested to explore or evaluate a particular organization against specified criteria. Here, the case is already decided, and research questions are then developed around the case. As shown in Figure 9.2, this situation is characteristic of an intrinsic study, the focus being on a particular case or cases.

At other times, perhaps prompted by an experience but responding to uncertainty over a more general situation, the researcher identifies research questions first. Theory may help guide the questions asked. Cases are subsequently selected. These questions are more characteristic of an instrumental or multiple case study because cases are selected to provide understanding of a wider situation (Stake, 1995).

Our research questions arose from experience. The International Classification of Functioning, Disability, and Health (ICF) (World Health Organization, 2001) shaped the way we asked the questions. The ICF defined participation as "involvement in a life situation" (World Health Organization, 2001, p. 10) and sees it as resulting not only from people's conditions such as TBI but also from their environment and life experience. Drawing on the ICF, the research questions were as follows:

From the perspectives of key stakeholders, for New Zealand children who have had a clinically significant TBI,

1   what aspects of their participation are important and
2   what are the facilitators and barriers to their participation?

Developing the conceptual framework

The next step in undertaking a case study is working out a conceptual framework. This initially provides a sound foundation for the study, then, as the study progresses, it gives a basis against which revised understandings may be articulated. The process of developing a conceptual framework involves three key stages: (1) developing issue statements and definitions, (2) delineating the case, and (3) developing topical questions.

Issue statements and definitions

Building on the research questions and drawing on researcher experience and theoretical understandings, issue statements (sometimes called propositions) may be developed (Simons, 2009; Stake, 1995, 2006; Yin, 2009). For example, guided by Margaret's experience, the ICF, and occupational therapy theory, the following issue statement was made in our study: "Physical, social, cultural, and institutional aspects of participation environments will be perceived by stakeholders to be either facilitators or barriers to the children's participation". This outlined the different aspects of the environment that we expected to either positively or negatively influence what the children did. The terms relating to the environment were defined, as were facilitators and barriers. Issue statements bring to the fore prior assumptions, suggest likely areas of concern, and, importantly, provide a conceptual base on which the next stages of the study are built. As such, issue statements often undergo revisions in response to findings as the study progresses.

Delineating the case

Texts highlight the importance of defining the case or "unit of analysis" (Yin, 2009, p. 29). This step involves establishing the various components of a case, so that its boundaries are clear and there is control over the scope of the project. Each case in our study was delineated as a New Zealand child with TBI and stakeholders who were involved with that child, such as family, teachers, and rehabilitation providers. A case also included the child's local community, and rehabilitation legislation and policy.

Different design features are considered at this point in the process. Options include the number of cases used and whether cases will have embedded units of analysis (i.e., subcases contained within them). When adopting an interpretive approach to the study, the number of cases is guided by the degree to which they provide for diversity or similarity. Depth of understanding about the phenomenon and its interactions with the context is also sought. Stake (2006) recommended that at least four cases are used for a multicase study. A decision was initially made to use five cases for our study, this number providing for diversity among children, their families, and settings, but still giving adequate depth of information within available time frames. As the study evolved, a sixth case was recruited to enhance understandings of long-term participation difficulties.

Developing topical questions

Issue statements, from stage 1, are used to generate specific topics. The topics then help with specifying the information that will be sought and lead to topical questions. To keep track of the multiple components we needed to consider, we developed a topical outline table (Stake, 1995;) (Table 9.1). Our table displayed topics in relation to the different components of the case which would serve as data sources. It pinpointed where information was triangulated across different components and highlighted any gaps. Items that we added later as understandings of the issues evolved were italicized. Aided by the table, specific topical questions were articulated which captured the information required from each component. The topical questions then supported development of interview and observation outlines. For example, a topical question that was integrated into all interview outlines was "How has the context of the participation changed?"

Table 9.1 Excerpt from topical outline and sources of information table

Issue statement Number	*1, 2, 3*	*3*	*3*	*3*
Primary and secondary topics for attention	*Description of participation context: home, school, community X physical, social, cultural, institutional + changes*	*Observed features of environment that facilitate/ limit participation and action/ modality*	*Perceived things that are facilitators to participation – How do they facilitate?*	*Perceived things that are barriers to participation – How do they limit?*
Data source and perspectives				
Child perspective	✓ + *changes*		✓	✓
Parent Perspective	✓ + *changes*		✓	✓
Teacher Perspective	✓ + *changes*		✓	✓
Observations	✓ (Description only)	✓	*(How only)*	*(How only)*
Doc. Analysis from Patient File	✓	✓	✓	✓

Case selection

As discussed earlier, although a case may have already been identified, on other occasions cases are selected purposively. Selection needs to ensure that participants in a case will meet the specified inclusion criteria, that they will generate answers to the topical questions, and that they provide adequate diversity or similarity between cases. People's availability and the location of the case also influence selection, given that data collection may extend over months. Once a case is selected, recruitment follows a process, as each case may involve several different participants.

Our study commenced with recruiting children and their parents. Criteria for children to be included as cases were that they were 9- to 12-year-olds, had sustained a moderate to severe TBI, had been discharged from inpatient settings at least 6 months previously, and were living in the community with their parent(s). Rehabilitation providers were enlisted to approach parents of children meeting the inclusion criteria. Parents who consented to take part then provided contact details for other important participants, such as teaching staff or rehabilitation case managers, and identified important activities which should be observed. In this way, participants played a part in shaping the case and immediately began identifying what was important about the children's participation.

Data collection

Project management

Before commencing data collection for a case study, a project management plan should be developed to ensure that data are gathered systematically and that the project overall runs smoothly. Plans detail information such as the conceptual structure and ethical approvals. They specify recruitment processes, participant contact details, safety procedures, equipment, and the sequencing of interviews and observations. Strategies for data analysis and a proposed outline for the case study report assist focus and preparedness for subsequent phases of the project (Stake, 1995; Yin, 2009).

Data sources

Case studies are characterized by the use of multiple data sources. This supports trustworthiness and gives diversity and breadth of information, particularly useful if the study is exploratory and new understandings are sought. Our data sources included a demographic questionnaire, interviews, observations, photographs of items, and rehabilitation documents.

Interviews

Semistructured interviews with children and family members took place at their homes while interviews with teaching staff occurred at school. An interview outline was used by Margaret to ensure information was generated that related to the topical questions. However, she remained responsive to participants' need to focus on particular aspects, as this often revealed unanticipated information about the children's participation. As data collection progressed, interview questions were informed by topics emerging from earlier data.

Given the level of involvement with people in each case across multiple contexts and time points, it was helpful to first establish rapport with participants. We found that by moving from the introduction on to some discussion of the accident, or to the first time of people's contact with the child, a start point was provided for their perceptions of participation changes or concerns.

For children, rapport was established by giving them a camera to take photos of objects that related to important occupations they engaged in. Interviews were then undertaken in the context of a poster-making occupation which incorporated the photos. Given the children experienced some communication difficulties, the challenge was to allow them time to answer and to avoid leading them to particular responses.

Observations

In gathering observational data, we were guided by parents' views as to which of their children's occupations were important. A participant observer role was adopted, which meant interacting naturally with people. This stance was supported because children's participation across settings typically involved the presence of several other adults, such as therapists or aides. Participant observations contrast with passive observations, which might have drawn more attention and resulted in behavior changes. Guided by the observation outline we had previously developed, brief notes were recorded during each occupation about the children's actions and interactions, and the contexts in which these occurred. The notes were written up in full, narrative style following the session. Observations generated rich data about the context of children's participation.

Document review

On the basis of information needs identified in the topical outline, copies of children's most recent rehabilitation documents were obtained. We were interested in the content, and the templates used, given these provide a context for the content. Documents particularly reflected the perspectives of rehabilitation providers and policy. These perspectives were often different to those of educators or parents but did not always capture aspects of participation observed in the community. For some cases, it was evident that rehabilitation perspectives had influenced parents' views about what was important. Direct influences of rehabilitation on children's participation were also apparent.

Data analysis

Given the variety of data collected with case study methodology, data analysis requires careful decisions about which analytic approach to use. In general, the process involves systematically breaking the data down into parts, discovering the meaning of those parts, then piecing them back together in a way that makes sense of the whole phenomenon and its context, and which provides answers to the research questions.

Common aspects of data analysis include in-depth description of the case and its context, preliminary interpretation of the data and coding, identification of patterns and connections in the coding, and development of assertions, or propositions. Where there are several cases, a cross-case analysis may be performed. Throughout the process, researchers must consider alternative interpretations while keeping a focus on the issues. However, different approaches to analysis vary according to the theoretical perspectives guiding the study, the types of questions an approach is designed to answer, and the degree to which the analysis is directed by the issue statements.

The research questions in our study reflected a need to learn and explore. Analysis was therefore guided by Stake's (1995) approach which aims to build understanding. This approach sees the researcher moving intuitively between direct interpretation of single instances of phenomena and aggregation of instances, weaving meaning both inductively and deductively to connect the parts with the whole (Dewey, 1910; Stake, 1995). Where there is repetition, patterns and relationships begin to suggest themselves. Data may be methodically searched for instances that either refute or confirm patterns and relationships.

Despite the guidance in Stake's text (1995), we found that the amount and diversity of the data was perplexing. Dewey's pragmatist philosophy acknowledged the need to explore all the different components of a situation but reminded us never to forget the continuity between people and context (1925/1981). We were concerned that by focusing on interpreting instances, and aggregating instances to find patterns (Stake, 1995), we risked losing sight of the whole picture. A mapping strategy was adopted (Simons, 2009), which enabled us to capture detail in the data across different data sources and to simultaneously make connections and comparisons, promoting a holistic view of each case in continuity with its contexts.

First, the interview transcripts, observation narratives, and documents were read methodically. Notations were made as to the meaning and what was happening. Names which conveyed the content of each chunk were allocated, these deriving from the data itself or from its suggested meaning. Data were considered in chunks rather than word by word to ensure the meaning was interpreted in context. However, where a word seemed significant, it was noted and its meaning considered in relation to the context of what was being said. For example, in Tish's case study, his parents explained that he was always first out of the school gate in the afternoon. His mother was asked "maybe the teacher lets him out first?" but she responded "No, I doubt it. She treats him just like everyone else . . . She doesn't want to spoil him or anything". The chunk of data was tentatively coded as 'Pace' noting Tish's speed, but after reflection, was re-coded as 'Being Treated the Same', noting it may involve not singling a child out or not indulging him.

The coded information for each participant or data source was mapped freely by hand onto individual sheets of semitransparent paper (the reason for which will become apparent below), using different colors to reflect each source. Brief direct quotes and their page numbers were incorporated to help capture the features of codes and to provide an audit trail. This process was intuitive, responding to the meanings interpreted from the data. Where codes seemed to be related to each other, arrows were drawn, and codes that seemed to have some similar qualities were situated nearby to each other, suggesting possible categories. For instance, Tish's father talked about his son's resistance to getting back into his school routines after the holidays, saying "I won't pamper it. You know we won't pamper it". This was coded as "Won't Pamper", with a note that it may reflect not giving special treatment and was situated next to the "Being Treated the Same" code. Data about the context were not seen as separate but were coded onto the map along with information about the child, to preserve the notion of a whole, continuous system.

With each new data source in a case, a different map was begun, semivisible below earlier maps (hence the value in using semitransparent paper). Efforts were made with these new data sources to craft the maps afresh. However, where codes were in line with those from earlier data sources, they were placed in a similar position on the new map. Illustrating this, it was noted that Tish, his teacher, his teacher aide, and observation records all discussed the importance of him being treated by adults and his peers in the same way as other children. The codes were also all situated next to things people did to help him fit in and be part of things, such as "Keeping an Eye on Him", "Welcoming", and "Seeking and Giving Help". This pattern was noted, and the group of codes across data sources were collectively called "Inclusive Actions".

In time, out of the mapping process, a model was derived that captured the patterns in the data and conveyed the important aspects of participation. The model varied slightly from case to case in terms of the categories included. The model that emerged from Tish's case is presented in Figure 9.3.

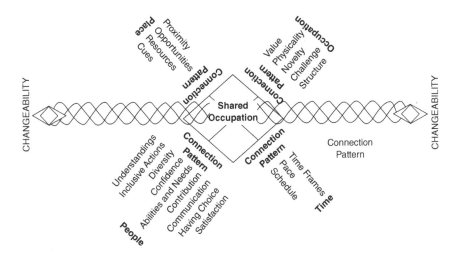

Figure 9.3 Model describing important aspects of Tish's participation

The central twisted lines represent the way children's participation was intertwined with others in their family and community. Arrows at either end indicate how participation was influenced by both the past and the future. Sharing in occupations together was central to participation, creating patterns across and connecting people, their occupations, places, and time. Potential and actual change in people, their occupations, place, and time was important; where there was too much or too little changeability, shared occupation was hampered. Equally, sharing in occupations was a means of prompting change, through people learning how to participate with each other (Textbox 9.2).

Textbox 9.2   The concepts in the model were illustrated during a kapa haka (traditional Māori dance) performance

Families have traveled many miles to see their children perform. . . . On stage the children's moves are polished. Younger children with less ability are merged, or positioned slightly behind, but incorporated into the group, others with skill carrying them through if a move is missed. There are poi songs, led by the girls, and innovative haka, performed by bare-chested boys with fearsome faces. The ground shakes with their stamping. Tish performs a dance with a spear – his performance is awesome – flawless and strikingly confident. I remember his mother telling me how last time . . . he just froze – no confidence. It's hard to believe now.

The narrative shows the way children and families were connected by sharing in an occupation at a point in time, and in a particular place. The occupation was changeable, with people adjusting children's positions on stage to embrace diversity, such as children's skill differences. With a pattern of regular participation in kapa haka, the children learned how to perform the movements and ways to support those with less ability to take part. Skill and confidence resulted for Tish.

Developing assertions

A further level of analysis may be undertaken in relation to the research questions by developing concluding statements about the case or cases (Simons, 2009). Stake (1995, p. 86) referred to these statements as "propositional generalizations" or "assertions". In developing assertions for our own study, mapped data from each source were searched for themes and processes that drew the children toward or away from participation (facilitators and barriers in the research question). Themes from each map were then integrated and overlaid onto the model (Figure 9.3), trying out different combinations and names until the themes were adequately captured. The assertions were framed by Dewey's (1938/2008) conceptualization of problematic situations and the practical solutions people determine to overcome them.

In Tish's case, a code of "restriction" was present across all data sources. People understood a risk of serious consequences from repeat concussion and acted by restricting his participation in valued physical occupations such as rugby to ensure his safety. Counteracting the restriction, several themes were found that involved people making changes to bring about new ways for him to participate. To draw the ideas together, the following assertions were stated:

> ***Qualifying the Problematic Situation: Restricted:*** Tish's participation was bound by the safety limits people placed on him.

> ***Determining Solutions: Finding New Ways:*** When people developed ways to change an occupation for Tish, created new, safer roles for him, or helped him learn new ways to perform an occupation, his participation was supported.

Case study report

Presenting case study findings is an important part of the methodology. A report may be informed by the original conceptual framework but will also reflect new discoveries and assertions that were developed. Reports can include any combination of narrative, direct quotations, diagrams, and quantitative data. They should provide vicarious experience of the case, therefore the audience must be kept in mind when developing the format.

In writing reports for each of our cases, the need to convey meaning clearly and concisely was balanced against providing depth of experience and meaning for readers. We anticipated that readers may be busy occupational therapists or families, so where possible, visual media such as photographs and diagrams were incorporated. Descriptions of themes and relationships drew on excerpts from the transcripts, communicating findings wherever possible in the words of the participants.

Data management

As with many qualitative studies, large amounts of data are generated and an organized approach to data management is essential. Based on our experiences, tips for managing data in a case study research are included in Textbox 9.3 below.

Textbox 9.3 Tips for case study data management

1   Focus on one case at a time.
2   For each case, keep a small, hard-cover notebook (labeled with your contact details) to record observations. Use pseudonyms. Write up observations promptly.
3   When analyzing confidential documents, remove identifiers first (we used a black felt pen), then photocopy, and work from the copies.

> 4   Identify all data with the case pseudonym and/or number, data source, and date of data collection. Number the pages.
>
> 5   For each case have a folder on your computer, and a large storage box for hard copies of analyzed data.
>
> 6   Use of color helps to keep track of the different data sources for each case during analysis.
>
> 7   Record and date actions, reflections, and decisions.

Rigor

The first strategy supporting rigor for a case study is clear articulation of the conceptual framework (Mitchell, 2000), which makes transparent the decisions undertaken at different stages in the research process. It demonstrates the connections between the research questions, the theoretical perspectives underlying the study, the issue statements, and the types of data sought from various data sources. In this way, readers can be assured of the logic underpinning the design.

Another feature of case studies that supports rigor is their iterative design. Decisions and interpretations are questioned in light of new data, experiences, emergent understandings, and existing theory. Alternative interpretations are reflected upon. New avenues for data collection may be sought. The researcher therefore looks back as well as forward, changing and refining the conceptual framework, plan, or interpretations where indicated. Such changes are reasoned (Yin, 2009), and the rationale is documented in an audit trail.

Case study research necessitates the close involvement of the researcher with multiple aspects of the case. Although efforts may be made not to unduly influence the data, ultimately researchers are closely connected with their cases, shaping the data gathered, its interpretation, and choices about what is most important to convey. A well-conducted case study will allow the reader to perceive the position of the researcher in relation to the data, and to weigh up for themselves the value of the interpretation and assertions generated.

Case studies often draw on multiple data sources and data collection strategies. While these provide depth of understanding and different perspectives about phenomena, through triangulation, they are also a means of confirming findings (Simons, 2009; Stake, 1995; Yin, 2009). The use of alternative theoretical perspectives, to explore study findings and member checking, further support reader trust in the study findings.

Most importantly, a rigorous case study conveys the case to the readers in detail rich enough to support vicarious experience. Where assertions are made, data should be provided and explained, so that readers can clearly see the path which led to those conclusions and also consider different interpretations. These strategies further enable readers to reflect on the way the case study information relates to their existing experiences and their understandings about phenomena, providing a foundation for learning. The degree to which information can be applied beyond the scope of the case study can be judged.

Ethics

In conducting a case study, researchers tread a fine line between portraying an accurate picture of the whole case and protecting anonymity of the participants. Careful choices therefore need to be made about which identifying details can safely be changed without compromising the integrity of the findings. Dilemmas can be posed within a case, where one participant expresses a view that may be hurtful or offensive to another participant. The first duty of the researcher is to ensure the well-being of the study participants, and data must be discarded if it cannot be used safely.

Specific ethical issues relating to the involvement of children with disabilities, informed consent, and the use of case files need to be addressed. Parents were requested to talk to their child about the study guided by a children's information sheet. If parents indicated they and their child were willing to take part, the children's understanding of the study was checked before formally seeking their verbal or signed consent and that of their parents. Specific consent was sought from children and parents to access case files

Critiquing case studies

Given the diverse applications of case study methodology, it is important to approach case study research with a critical eye. Any critique must first recognize a study's theoretical underpinnings, which bear influence on the design and findings. Questions that can guide critical appraisal of a case study are listed in Textbox 9.4.

Textbox 9.4 Critiquing case studies – questions to ask

1 Are the *theoretical perspectives* of the case study clearly stated and justified?
2 Is the *role of the researcher* in relation to the study clearly articulated?
3 Does the description of the *conceptual framework* show clear linkages from the question and theoretical perspectives to the types and sources of data sought?
4 Has the case been clearly defined?
5 Was the *safety and anonymity* of the participants assured?
6 Were the strategies used for data collection and analysis systematic, clearly described, and justified?
7 Is there evidence that the research process was *responsive to unexpected events* or findings?
8 Were changes to the original protocol justified and reasonable?
9 Were *alternative explanations* for findings sought and discussed?
10 Is the *context* of the case adequately described and integrated with the findings?

11 Is the case study report rich, engaging, and accessible for its readers?
12 Is the case cohesive, with *findings and assertions* considered in relation to the original questions and theoretical understandings?
13 Is it clear how the *assertions or propositions* were derived? Do they make sense in relation to other information in the study?
14 Does the case study *provide new insights* into the issue?

Application to occupational science

This is one of the few studies exploring participation in occupations for school-age children after occupational disruption resulting from a traumatic event such as a TBI. The adoption of a case study methodology meant that the environment was integral to the project, enabling a range of perspectives to be gained in some depth. The contextual situation of people's occupations is well recognized in occupational science literature. This study contributed to understandings about the interrelationships between children's contexts and their participation, and how those relationships influence the quality of participation.

The study found that for these children, sharing occupations with others was fundamental to participation. The quality of shared occupation was reflected in the patterns and connections formed across different people, their occupations, places, and times. As the children and others around them participated in shared occupations, they changed, gaining understandings and skills that furthered their ability to participate with others. The degree to which a child and context underwent change was an important influence; too much or too little change hampered participation in shared occupations, creating a negative spiral, where the lack of participation further blocked change and learning about how to participate.

Application to occupational therapy

In highlighting the centrality of shared occupation to participation, and the learning of participation skills, the study draws occupational therapy practitioners' attention to the importance of the social environment. Disrupted participation as a result of injury, extensive participation in rehabilitation, and prevention of participation due to ongoing safety concerns can create a cycle where lack of shared occupation hampers the child's, their peers', and others' learning in the community about how to participate with each other.

The findings highlight the shortcomings of interventions for children's participation after a TBI, which have typically been directed at the child and aspects of his or her occupational performance. Strategies that immediately promote shared occupation, and which enable children and their peers to learn how to participate with each other, are needed to facilitate participation.

Personal reflections

With our natural tendency to view occupation as both complex and contextualized, we were drawn to case study methodology by its ability to tease out the particulars of a person's occupations while maintaining continuity with the whole of their world. As we completed the case study, we looked afresh at what we knew before we began and what was revealed by the project. The conceptual structure was like an imprint on a backing fabric, against which each case was formed and bordered. Moving backward and forward between the parts of the case and the bigger picture, what initially seemed confusing began to make sense and patterns began to form. Sometimes, we needed to attend to a small detail, critical to building understanding, other times we stepped back and looked at the design as a whole. With frequent reference to texts, and support from those with more experience, confidence was slowly gained. Together with the participants, we have depicted the children's participation in their New Zealand context, methodically pieced together to share with, and to be of use to, others.

Conclusion

Tish's experience of being told he could not participate in rugby, an occupation he valued and enjoyed before his injury, was repeated across the cases completed in our study. That experience informed one of our key findings, that children's participation is supported when others have skills in driving their engagement, by visioning, learning about, weighing up, planning for, preparing for, and pressing them toward shared occupation. That might involve taking on a role of leading others and actively including the children. When those leadership skills are lacking and children's capacity for occupation does not fit the demands, they miss out on opportunities for development. Our choice of case study methodology was crucial in reaching those understandings, because of the importance placed on gathering data from multiple viewpoints and paying attention to contextual influences. From our perspective, that is exactly what is required to understand the complexities of occupation, as a phenomenon embedded in the messiness of people's everyday lives.

Acknowledgments

To the Health Research Council of New Zealand for funding support.

References

Cameron, D., Cockburn, L., Nixon, S., Parnes, P., Garcia, L., Leotaud, J., . . . Williams, T. (2013). Global partnerships for international fieldwork in occupational therapy: Reflection and innovation. *Occupational Therapy International, 20*(2), 88–96. doi:10.1002/oti.1352.

Cresswell, J. W. (2007). *Qualitative inquiry and research design: Choosing among five approaches* (2nd ed.). Thousand Oaks, CA: Sage.

Cutchin, M. P., & Dickie, V. A. (Eds.). (2013). *Transactional perspectives on occupation.* New York, NY: Springer. doi:10.1007/978-94-007-4429-5.

Darragh, A. R., Campo, M. A., Frost, L., Miller, M. L., Pentico, M., & Margulis, H. (2013). Safe-patient-handling equipment in therapy practice: Implications for rehabilitation. *American Journal of Occupational Therapy, 67*, 45–53. doi:10.5014/ajot.2013.005389.

Dewey, J. (1910). *How we think.* Retrieved from http://archive.org/stream/howwethink 000838mbp#page/n13/mode/2up

Dewey, J. (1916). *Democracy and education: An introduction to the philosophy of education.* Retrieved from http://en.wikisource.org/wiki/Democracy_and_Education

Dewey, J. (1925/1981). Experience and nature. In J. A. Boydston (Ed.), *John Dewey: The later works, 1925–1953: (Volume 1).* Carbondale, IL: Southern Illinois University Press.

Dewey, J. (1938/2008). Logic: The theory of inquiry. In J. A. Boydston (Ed.), *John Dewey: The later works, 1925–1953: (Volume 12).* Carbondale, IL: Southern Illinois University Press.

Donnelly, C., Brenchley, C., Crawford, C., & Letts, L. (2013). The integration of occupational therapy into primary care: A multiple case study design. *BMC Family Practice, 14*, 60. doi:10.1186/1471-2296-14-60.

Gerring, J. (2007). *Case study research: Principles and practices.* New York, NY: Cambridge University Press.

Hammersly, M., & Gomm, R. (2000). Introduction. In R. Gomm, M. Hammersley, & P. Foster (Eds.), *Case study method: Key issues, key texts* (pp. 1–16). London, UK: Sage.

Hesse-Biber, S. N., & Leavy, P. (2011). *The practice of qualitative research* (2nd ed.). Thousand Oaks, CA: Sage.

Ilott, I., Kottorp, A., la Cour, K., van Nes, F., Jonsson, H., & Sadlo, G. (2013). Sustaining international partnerships: The European Master of Science Programme in Occupational Therapy: A case study. *Occupational Therapy International, 20*(2), 55–64. doi:10.1002/oti.134.

Merriam, S. B. (2009). *Qualitative research: A guide to design and implementation* (Rev. ed.). San Francisco, CA: Jossey-Bass.

Mitchell, J. C. (2000). Case and situation analysis. In R. Gomm, M. Hammersley, & P. Foster (Eds.), *Case study method: Key issues, key texts* (pp. 165–186). London, UK: Sage.

Platt, J. (1992). "Case study" in American methodological thought. *Current Sociology, 40*, 17–48. doi:10.1177/001139292040001004.

Provident, I. M., & Comer, M. (2013). Muscular dystrophy summer camp: A case study of a non-traditional level I fieldwork using a collaborative supervision model. *WORK: A Journal of Prevention, Assessment & Rehabilitation, 44*, 337–404. doi:10.3233/WOR-121510.

Simons, H. (2009). *Case study research in practice.* London, UK: Sage.

Smith, Y. J., Stephenson, S., & Gibson-Satterthwaite, M. (2013). The meaning and value of traditional occupational practice: A Karen woman's story of weaving in the United States. *Work, 45*(1), 25–30. doi:10.3233/WOR-131600.

Stake, R. E. (1995). *The art of case study research.* Thousand Oaks, CA: Sage.

Stake, R. E. (2006). *Multiple case study analysis.* New York, NY: The Guilford Press.

World Health Organization. (2001). *International classification of functioning, disability and health (ICF).* Geneva, Switzerland: Author.

Yin, R. K. (2009). *Case study research: Design and methods* (4th ed.). Los Angeles, CA: Sage.

Further reading

Baxter, P., & Jack, S. (2008). Qualitative case study methodology: Study design and implementation for novice researchers. *The Qualitative Report, 13*(4), 544–559.

Websites

Gibbs, G. R. (2012). *Types of case study. Part 1 of 3 on case studies.* Retrieved from http://www.youtube.com/watch?v=gQfoq7c4UE4

Gibbs, G. R. (2012). *Planning a case study. Part 2 of 3 on case studies.* Retrieved from http://www.youtube.com/watch?v=o1JEtXkFAr4

Gibbs, G. R. (2012). *Replication or single cases. Part 3 of 3 on case studies.* Retrieved from http://www.youtube.com/watch?v=b5CYZRyOlys

Johansson, R. (2003, September). *Case study methodology.* Paper presented at the International Conference "Methodologies in Housing Research", Stockholm, Sweden. Retrieved from http://www.psyking.net/HTMLobj-3839/Case_Study_Methodology-_Rolf_Johansson_ver_2.pdf

10 Critical discourse analysis

Opening possibilities through deconstruction

Debbie Laliberte Rudman and Silke Dennhardt

Variants of discourse analysis, alone or in combination with other methodologies, are more frequently being used in occupation-focused research. Although examples of studies cover a range of substantive areas and research purposes, the focus on how discourses – that is, ways of writing and talking about a phenomena – shape possibilities for how groups of people can and do act in the world hold them together as studies employing discourse analysis. For example, Ballinger and Payne (2000b, 2002) combined critical discourse analysis and ethnography to interrogate how risk was understood and enacted in a community day hospital, pointing to how a dominant biomedical discourse on risk minimizes agency for older clients and positions health care professionals as experts. Johansson, Lilja, Park, and Josephsson (2010) combined critical discourse analysis and narrative inquiry to examine interactions between hegemonic organizational discourses and the practices of service providers in home modification services. Using variants of discourse analysis, Kantartzis and Molineux (2012) deconstructed assumptions about occupation that shape occupational science research, and Pereira (2013) interrogated social inclusion policy and its implications for occupations.

Within this chapter, we draw on our experiences of using a particular approach to discourse analysis, specifically, critical discourse analysis. Our shared research interest lies in enhancing understanding of how occupational possibilities become shaped within specific sociopolitical contexts; that is, how discourses contribute to "what people take for granted as what they can and should do, and the occupations that are supported and promoted by various aspects of the broader systems and structures in which their lives are lived" (Laliberte Rudman, 2010, p. 55). Both studies used as examples in this chapter employed critical discourse analysis informed by a governmentality theoretical perspective. The first study, referred to as the 'retirement study', examined the discursive construction of aging and retirement in media documents (Laliberte Rudman, 2005, 2006; Laliberte Rudman, Huot, & Dennhardt, 2009; Laliberte Rudman & Molke, 2009) to address how discourses, and the identity and occupational possibilities they promote, are taken up, resisted, and negotiated by aging individuals (Laliberte Rudman, 2013, 2014). The second study, referred to as the 'risky driver study', examined how risk is taken up to govern everyday occupation and focused on how risk was used within information brochures to constitute an ideal occupational subjectivity for aging drivers and outline practices for aging individuals to responsibly govern their driving (Dennhardt, 2013; Dennhardt & Laliberte Rudman, 2012).

Background: discourse analysis and critical discourse analysis

Discourse analysis is a broad methodological space, and debate exists regarding its defining features and what counts as a discourse analysis (Ballinger & Cheek, 2006). The diversity of approaches labeled discourse analysis stems from interdisciplinary origins and a multiplicity of theoretical and philosophical underpinnings. For example, definitions of discourse may refer to any instance of communication, language used in a particular field of practice, or to instances of talk or text that contain particular properties (Cheek, 2004; Fairclough, 2009). As for examples of diversity in research approaches, discourse analysis, as enacted in ethnomethodological research, is focused on how language is interactively used to organize social action within local contexts; for example, how communicative processes structure work within an occupational therapy clinic. Approaches located within discursive constructionism focus on how discourses are employed in interactions in ways that construct everyday reality, as well as the range of linguistic resources drawn upon to construct discourses (Holstein & Gubrium, 2011). Approaches informed by poststructural perspectives, often labeled critical discourse analysis, are concerned with how discourses enact power through shaping possibilities for being and acting and how subjects negotiate the self and everyday life in relation to discourses (Ainsworth & Hardy, 2004a, 2004b).

Given that discourse analysis is not a unified approach, we do not provide a singular definition nor attempt to address all of its diverse approaches. Rather, in this chapter, we focus on a particular variant of discourse analysis, specifically, critical discourse analysis, and address its potential contributions to the study of occupation and occupational therapy. We have chosen this focus because we see it as a valuable research methodology to advancing understanding of occupation as situated within various contextual conditions. It is important to clarify that critical discourse analysis is always framed by a theoretical framework (Wodak & Meyer, 2009), it is neither a fixed method nor a singular methodology but an approach to conceptualize and study discourse as a social practice. We strongly agree with Cheek (2004) that there cannot be a set of rules for critical discourse analysis and it is important to work against framing discourse analysis as "a value free technology – a theory free method and tool to do research" (p. 1148).

Epistemological assumptions and methodological implications

The addition of the word 'critical' to 'discourse analysis' signals the centrality of paradigmatic positioning (van Dijk, 2009). The use of the word critical refers to interlinked ontological and epistemological assumptions. Ontologically, critical discourse analysis studies are characterized by a position of tentative realism, in which social reality is viewed as 'reified' over time through interactions of social, political, economic, cultural, gender and other factors, in ways that particular structures and systems become taken as if they were real rather than socially constructed. Epistemologically, critically informed qualitative research-ers assume that language is key in the shaping of social life and in the enact-ment of power. Thus, how an object, such as mental health or a group of people, such as First Nations youth, is discursively constructed shapes the way systems, structures, processes, and practices are constructed and enacted in relation to that phenomenon (Mumby, 2004). The primacy placed on language leads to a focus on the form, content and structure of discourse, as well as an overarching aim to deconstruct the ways language is used to construct 'realities' about particular phenomenon and particular types of people.

Critical discourse analysis, as taken up in health sciences, has been greatly influenced by the theoretical work of Foucault, in addition to other poststructural perspectives (Cheek, 2004; Hardin, 2003). As such, definitions of discourse used within critical discourse analysis draw on a poststructural view of language as a social practice, emphasizing the productive, constitutive, and value-laden nature of language (Allen & Hardin, 2001; Ballinger & Cheek, 2006). As can be seen in Textbox 10.1, such definitions focus on discourses as systems of meaning, conveyed through talk and text, which produce particular versions of concepts, objects, and subject positions (Hardy & Phillips, 2004).

Textbox 10.1   Understanding discourse in critical discourse analysis – example definitions of discourse

"practices that systematically form the objects [and subjects] of which they speak" (Foucault, 1972, p. 49)

"broad social, cultural, and historical systems of meanings, creating both the notion of the 'self' and how the 'self' constructs its world" (Hardin, 2001, p. 14)

"chains of signifiers that orientate our behavior around a discursive object" (Allen & Hardin, 2001, p. 168)

"scaffolds of discursive frameworks, which order reality in a certain way. They both enable and constrain the production of knowledge, in that they allow for certain ways of thinking about reality while exclud-ing others" (Cheek, 2004, p. 1142)

Overall, definitions of discourse commensurate with critical discourse analysis refer to discourse as a productive social practice, intimately tied to power, that constructs what comes to be taken-for-granted as 'real' or 'truth' in a particular sociohistorical context (Mumby, 2004). What is essential is that rather than view-ing language as making visible an extra-linguistic reality (e.g., the meaning asso-ciated with an occupation), there is a focus on how meaning, subjectivities (e.g., 'the unemployed'), and objects are created in and through language (Ainsworth & Hardy, 2004a). This shifts the focus of analysis away from the individual and the meaning he or she assigns to an occupation toward situating individual accounts and occupations within broader discourses (Hardin, 2003). As an example, Allen and Hardin (2001) point to discourses of gender that outline constructions of men and women that include possibilities for their being and doing. In turn, individuals become men and women and reproduce social arrangements through repeating the language of such discourses and engaging in the occupational possibilities they promote.

In line with their critical position, various approaches to critical discourse analysis are concerned with the power effects of discourse; that is, the ways in which power is enacted by a range of social authorities and agencies through the discursive production of 'normalizing truths' (Allen & Hardin, 2001; Fairclough, 2009). Attending to such power effects, Hardy and Phillips (2004) explained that discourse both "'rules in' certain ways of talking about a topic" and "'rules out', limits and restricts other ways of talking, of conducting ourselves in relation to the topic or constructing knowledge about it" (p. 300). While realizing that there may be a number of discourses pertaining to any particular type of subject or object, there is a focus on the marginalizing and exclusionary effects of dominant discourses. For example, in the 'retirement study', we examined the ways in which the dominant discourse on ideal housing for retirement excluded aging individuals with significant physical or cognitive disabilities and those with inadequate financial resources to participate in the private housing market (Laliberte Rudman et al., 2009). Given that multiple, often competing, discourses exist, analysis can also attend to how people negotiate their possibilities for being and doing within the discourses accessible within their specific sociohistorical conditions (Hardin, 2003). For example, in the 'retirement study', the ways that individuals conveyed their stories of retirement were not taken as reflections of unmediated inner feelings or a core self. Rather the form and content of the narratives were examined in relation to how individuals actively drew upon and negotiated broader discourses of aging to shape themselves as subjects and make sense of their occupations (Laliberte Rudman, 2013, 2014).

Another key assumption is that discourses are themselves situated within relations of power (Wodak & Meyer, 2009). In turn, critical discourse analysis studies involve situating discourses within broader sociopolitical, economic, cultural, and other contextual forces (Holstein & Gubrium, 2011). For example, in both the retirement and risky driver study, we have found that dominant discourses emphasize individual responsibility through outlining what individuals should do to ensure health, autonomy, and other idealized outcomes. Situating this individualizing of responsibility within the broader contemporary sociopolitical context, we have pointed to ways dominant discourses on aging well and driving well align with the values and aims of neoliberalism (Dennhardt, 2013; Laliberte Rudman, 2006, 2013).

A further essential feature of critical discourse analysis is the commitment to a critical intent. Such an intent aims to address situations of injustice through challenging dominant rationalities and ideologies, questioning the taken-for-granted ways society has come to be structured, creating space for resistance and change, and raising awareness of how discourses shape disparities (Ballinger & Payne, 2000a; Wodak & Meyer, 2009). For example, in the retirement study, Debbie questioned the taken-for-granted 'positivity' of dominant discourses of 'positive' aging by examining how positive aging discourses have been taken up in ways that align with broader governmental aims to retreat from programs and services for aging citizens and limit spaces for occupation for certain types of aging subjects.

Research purposes and critical discourse analysis

Critical discourse analysis studies aim to raise awareness of how discourses shape possibilities for how people understand their worlds and themselves, as well as what they view as possible and ideal ways to be and do in everyday life. This methodological approach is an appropriate choice within research studies that aim to situate individual accounts of experiences, including occupations within broader social, political, economic, racial, and gendered contexts (Holstein & Gubrium, 2011). As articulated by Hardin (2003), critical discourse analysis enables a researcher to "move data beyond the level of the individual and into historical, social and cultural realms" (p. 544).

Research purposes that fit with critical discourse analysis encompass questioning the ways dominant discourses shape injustices and inequities (Ainsworth & Hardy, 2004b), including injustices and inequities related to occupation. For example, in the 'retirement study', one research purpose was to raise awareness of the ways in which assumptions about who older workers are and what types of work they should engage in constructed via dominant discourses of 'productive' aging may set up inequities between older and younger workers and among older workers. This translated into research questions such as: What types of subjectivities are presented within a contemporary Canadian media source as ideal and non-ideal for aging and older workers? What practices of the self are presented as ways to work toward achieving ideal subjectivities? What forms and types of work are presented as ideal and non-ideal for aging and older workers?

Constructing the research field

Since discourses are realized within and through texts (Fairclough, 1995), critical discourse analysis studies use texts as the data. Texts can include printed materials that 'pre-exist' (such as newspaper texts, governmental policies, or historical documents) or are produced in the research process (such as interview transcripts or photo diaries). 'Texts' are "any kind of symbolic expression requiring a physical medium and permitting of permanent storage" (Hardy & Philips, 2004, p. 300). Thus, depending on the research questions, various types of texts in which everyday discourses are (re)produced, such as toys (van Leeuwen, 2008), cartoons (Hardy & Phillips, 1999), games (Millington, 2011), or diagnostic manuals (DSM-IV) (Crowe, 2001), can be employed.

As in all qualitative research, the research field in critical discourse analysis "is not out there waiting to be described by researchers" (Cheek, 2000, p. 126) and does not exist independently from the researcher and the questions posed. A primary goal of data collection is to generate a data-rich body of texts that can be expected to offer new insights into how the social phenomenon under investigation is constituted (Phillips & Hardy, 2002). For instance, one rationale for choosing information brochures for aging drivers in the 'risky driver study' was that these texts are explicitly produced to address aging drivers. Thus, brochures were expected to contain rich data on how the occupational subjectivity of the aging driver is discursively constructed, given that texts which target a particular group of subjects need to discursively establish these subjects as somehow 'different' from the implicit main group (Castel, 1991).

Selecting and analyzing relevant texts are interwoven tasks that inform and build on each other. While gathering and selecting texts needs to be provisional and emergent in accordance with analysis, it is a systematic scholarly process, grounded in a study's research questions, theoretical framework, and methodology (Phillips & Hardy, 2002). Since discourses are not a pre-existing object that can be 'revealed' by investigating a particular number of texts, there is an awareness that researchers "can only trace clues to them regardless of how much data they collect" (Phillips & Hardy, 2002, p. 74). Therefore, the challenge of data collection is not to find 'all' possible texts 'out there', but rather to decide which texts to choose to best trace discourses of interest (Jäger & Maier, 2009; Phillips & Hardy, 2002).

Data analysis methods

Approaches to data analysis embrace a broad variety of analytic methods, with the process best described as an individualist approach that is creatively customized for each study to translate its theoretical underpinnings into productive analysis methods (Jørgensen & Phillips, 2002; Wodak & Meyer, 2009). In this section, we draw primarily on the risky driver study to illustrate the analysis process constructed and enacted.

Key features of analysis in critical discourse analysis

Integrating theory in analysis is essential in ensuring interpretations go beyond surface meanings (Phillips & Hardy, 2002; Wodak & Meyer, 2009). A strategy we both used to facilitate theory-informed data analysis is the development of an analysis sheet (Jäger & Maier, 2009; Richardson, 2007) (see Textbox 10.2 for an example). Besides their value in facilitating theory-informed analysis, we found that analysis sheets helped to ensure transparency of the analysis process and facilitated cross-text analysis.

Data analysis is an emergent process that is constantly refined in response to the overall research process and understandings of the analyzed data (Hardy & Phillips, 1999; Jørgensen & Phillips, 2002). Initially, the analysis sheet in the risky driver study did not contain questions related to the aging body. When it was found that the body was repeatedly mentioned across texts and constructed in relation to driving, a new set of questions were added to guide attention to the constructed relationship between driving and the body, self-body relationships, and the body as an object of governing.

Textbox 10.2   Examples of questions included in an analysis sheet

Analysis sheets guide a theory-informed reading that pushes beyond a text's superficial content and facilitates attending to its form and function in producing content, social meaning, and power relations (Fairclough, 1995). Such sheets contain guiding questions informed by (1) framing theory, (2) research questions, and (3) tools for deconstructing texts. Examples of questions from the 'risky driver' study:

1   informed by theory (here: governmentality):
    • Problematization: What is being problematized? Where is the problem located? What social problems are to be alleviated/what social goals are to be achieved? Power relations: Who is defining the problems? Who is proposing the solutions? Who is likely to benefit from the discourse?

2   informed by research questions (here: related to the occupation 'later life driving'):
    • Occupation: How is the occupation conceptualized in the text (e.g., As an individual or social occupation? As a 'right or privilege'? As a leisure activity?) Who engages in it and who does or should not? What is absent with regard to the way the occupation is constructed? What kind of relationship are subjects called to take toward their occupation?

3   informed by tools for deconstruction (here: critical linguistics, Richardson, 2007)
    • Naming and reference: How are subjects within the texts named and referred to? Which adjectives and pronouns (e.g., 'us' and 'they') are used? Which qualities, attributes, and characteristics (positive/negative?) are linguistically assigned? What subject positions, social relations and social values do the employed referential strategies construct?

A second key feature is that analysis is multilayered, employing and combining multiple level and foci of analysis (Fairclough, 1995; Jäger & Maier, 2009). Approaches to data analysis include various methods of 'deconstruction' and the use of linguistic tools (Richardson, 2007; Wodak & Meyer, 2009). Deconstructive approaches involve a certain way of reading and investigating texts, which does not aim to find the meaning within a text nor to reveal an assumed underlying 'truth'. Rather, deconstruction aims to expose and 'unsettle' implicit meanings and assumptions, including a text's taken-for-granted perspectives, categorizations, binary oppositions, its absences, and so on (Cheek, 2000). For instance, analysis investigates presuppositions that a sentence such as 'Make transportation an important consideration in choosing a retirement home' contains – such as, that aging subjects have the possibility to 'choose' a retirement home, that it is 'normal' and expected to move to a retirement home at one point in one's future, and that subjects can shape their future mobility positively by 'making' it important and preparing for it.

Given that a text's content is never independent of its form and organization, analysis needs to attend to both what is said and the 'texture' of texts (Fairclough, 1995). Thus, the use of linguistic tools and concepts, such as syntax, mode, tense, actors, grammar, vocabulary and so forth, is essential (Richardson, 2007). Textual analysis in the risky driver study closely attended to how subjects were linguistically categorized and separated (e.g., 'most older drivers, as a *sign of continued good judgment*', 'other drivers *stubbornly deny*') and how referential strategies functioned in constructing ideal and nonideal subject positions (such as the subjectivity of a self-aware, responsible, 'safe' individual versus the subjectivity of an inflexible, denying, and risky 'other').

Analysis of the form and organization of printed text also attends to a text's visual elements such as layout, headings, images, symbols, and colors, attending to interrelationships between visual and other textual material. For example, in the risky driver study, accompanying images, which encompassed photos, cartoon-like, and sketchy drawings, shared many similarities (Textbox 10.3). These recurring images were interpreted as functioning together with printed text; they employed similar discursive strategies, such as the use of biomedical expertise to shape aging bodies as inherently risky, the emphasis on personal responsibility for oneself and others, and the promotion of healthy aging as a means to continue safe driving.

Textbox 10.3   Example of attending to visual images

Through systematically noting features of images included in information brochures for aging drivers, repetitive features were identified. These included

- *an image of a medical scene*, object, or symbol, such as pill containers, a stethoscope, or a woman getting an eye examination
- *an image of a driving scene, often a potentially dangerous one*, such as a cluttered traffic scene, a busy intersection, or a night scene
- *an image of individuals positioned close to each other*, implying a caring and loving relationship, such as images of couples and families, standing close to each other, resting the arm on another individual's shoulder, or one individual looking at another

- *an image showing or signifying an active and healthy lifestyle,* such as, an aging individual riding a bike or holding an apple
- *an image emphasizing an individual as a driver,* such as a person holding a key or behind the wheel; or an image taken from the inside of a car to the outside, positioning the reader within the car and as the driver
- *an image showing or signifying transportation other than driving,* such as a shuttle-bus or a bus pass
- *an educational or symbolic image,* such as a vehicle with suggested safety features, or a green and red traffic light, pointing to a 'good' practice to take up or a 'bad' one to avoid

Another important focus for textual analysis in critical discourse analysis is attending to absences (Fairclough, 1995; Wood & Kroger, 2000); that is, examining the text in terms of "what is present and what *could* have been but is *not* present" (Richardson, 2007, p. 38, emphasis in original). By drawing out what is recurrently absent when texts frame a particular social issue, analysis can address how dominant problem frames exclude alternative ways of thinking about and approaching an issue. For example, in the risky driver study, attending to absences enabled identification of the relative neglect of solutions to the 'aging driver problem' that focused on societal actions, as opposed to individual actions.

As analysis proceeds, different level and foci of analysis are analytically related to each other (Fairclough, 1995; Jørgensen & Phillips, 2002). In the risky driver study, continually writing analytical notes ensured connections were made between different level and foci. In addition to recording impressions, insights, or data-rich quotations on analysis sheets, analytical and reflexive notes were written. These notes took different forms, such as free writing, summarizing first insights across texts, or drawing visual understandings. Form and foci of notes altered as analysis moved from early to later cycles. For instance, earlier cycles of analysis involved more free and open notes about ideas that came to mind, while later notes focused on systematically putting things together and linking different foci of analysis.

The process of analysis

The analytic process is iterative, interwoven, and nonlinear (Jäger & Maier, 2009). Thus, while described separately, the main cycles of analysis in the risky driver study were repeated several times, sometimes separate from each other and sometimes in parallel, ultimately overlapping and feeding into each other in many ways. Main cycles of analysis included open reading, theory-informed reading, and textual analysis within single texts, as well as cross-text analysis and contextualizing findings.

Within-text analysis began with an open reading of a text, accompanied by free note writing. First notes were broad and contained various initial impressions, and reactions, referring to various textual levels (i.e., form, function, content). To not constrain potential interpretation early in the analytical process, these initial notes attended more to "the possibility that something interesting was going on, rather than [to] an indication of what it might be" (Wood & Kroger, 2000, p. 92). Open reading also included a careful 'reading' of semiotic elements included in the text, such as photographs, checkmarks, or self-tests. For instance, in 'reading' a photograph for the first time in the risky driver study, any detail of the picture was described (e.g., 'good teeth', 'white hair', 'woman looking up'). Though at times tedious, this strategy of detailed description facilitated stepping outside taken-for-granted 'ways of seeing' (Rose, 2007) and enhanced analysis profoundly.

Next, the text was read again, using a theory-informed lens. Focused reading, informed by governmentality, was guided by questions on the analysis sheet, such as "Who is defining the problem and who is addressed as having power to 'fix' it?" and "What practices of the self are the targeted audience called upon to participate in?" Such theory-informed analysis enabled another level of critical reading.

Each text was also read 'linguistically', focusing on how particular meanings were created by form and function features. For instance, particular types of verb choices which were consistently repeated within and across texts were marked. Texts repeatedly called upon aging subjects to 'remain', 'stay', and 'continue' to be safe drivers, as well as to 'maintain', 'preserve', and 'keep' their body's driving fitness. Applying linguistic tools, these verbs were investigated with regard to what presuppositions and meanings these particular verb choices shared (i.e., these verbs imply that something involuntarily worsens or is lost if nobody takes action to maintain it), where in a text they were primarily used (i.e., these verbs are dominantly used when safety or the aging body is brought up), and how actors and objects were linguistically related. The findings of this cycle of analysis (i.e., these verbs stress that one has to work actively against an underlying process to 'keep' one's status) were then combined with previous and later findings of other cycles and foci of analysis, such as when analysis demonstrated how driving and the aging body become constructed as risk objects in need for self-governing.

The second main cycle of analysis contained cross-text analysis in which texts were repeatedly read 'against' each other. Analysis in this cycle focused on similarities, variations, contrasts, repetitions, connections, contradictions, and absences in content, form, and function across texts. For instance, early on in the process it was noticed that almost all texts in the risky driver study contained numerical representations, such as measures of declining body function or accident statistics. Systematically investigating this observation showed that quantification techniques served similar functions across texts; for example, establishing age-related changes in body function and driving ability as objective, calculable and predictable 'facts' which are measurable and thus 'truly' existing. Moreover, quantification techniques, by mainly drawing upon biomedical knowledges, also constructed driving as an individual occupation and the problems associated with the occupation as solely located in aging bodies and irresponsible body 'owners' – and not, for example, in an autocentered organization of space, time, and social relations.

Rigor

Within the field of critical discourse analysis, there is no consensus regarding quality criteria (Wodak & Meyer, 2009). Given its epistemological assumptions, critical discourse analysis does not aim to produce the most 'accurate' reading. Rather it aims to produce a reading that draws upon theory to question taken-for-granted assumptions and related practices (Cheek, 2004).

In our work, we have found the four considerations outlined by Ballinger (2006) to be helpful in addressing quality issues when enacting a critical discourse analysis. These considerations include coherence, systematic and careful research conduct, convincing and relevant interpretation, and accounting for the role of researchers. Coherence, referring to the overall fit between the elements of a study, such as its theoretical frame, research objectives, and analytical foci, is particularly crucial given that critical discourse analysis is always theoretically framed. For this to be appraised, it is essential that the theoretical grounding is made explicit from the beginning of a study, and the ways in which it is drawn upon to frame the study is articulated (Wodak & Meyer, 2009).

Systematic and careful research conduct is demonstrated through careful documentation, such as a decision trail, that supports the plausibility and persuasiveness of the interpretative analysis (Ballinger, 2006; Cheek, 2004). The ultimate evaluation of the extent to which a study is convincing and relevant, Ballinger's third quality consideration, resides in the reader. A relevant critical discourse analysis should offer a new reading of texts through drawing on theoretical perspectives and address the structures, strategies, and situatedness of discourses. "Indeed, the whole point should be to provide insights into structures, strategies or other properties of discourse that could not readily be given by naïve recipients" (van Dijk, 1997, p. 5).

A fourth consideration is the need to account for the role of the researcher, noting that this is often done through reflexivity (Ballinger, 2006). Reflexive researchers provide their audience with information about themselves and their perspectives and engage in practices to reflect on their own subjectivities and their discursive positioning. As such, researchers need to be aware that their own work is shaped within a specific sociopolitical context and thus must be explicit regarding the values that inform what they define as situations of injustice and inequity (Wodak & Meyer, 2009).

To conclude this section, we provide a set of critical questions in Textbox 10.4 that we have found helpful to guide appraisal of the quality of a critical discourse analysis.

**Textbox 10.4   Reviewing critical discourse analysis studies –
questions to ask**

1   Do the researchers locate the study epistemologically and provide
information about a *theoretical framework* that informs their critical
discourse analysis?

2   Do the researchers provide a *definition of discourse* and is their definition congruent with the study's theoretical framework?

3   Are *language choices* within the article in line with the underlying
theory?

4   Do the authors provide a rationale for how the *body of texts was constructed*? Does their choice of texts enable them to address the study's
research question?

5   Do the authors *systematically outline the strategies* used to search for
and/or produce texts, as well as the criteria used to include and exclude
texts?

6   Does the analysis pay attention to both *what is said* (content) and *how it
is said*? Commensurate with the theoretical framework employed, does
the analysis attend to the *potential effects* of particular discourses (e.g.,
identity possibilities, occupational possibilities)?

7   Are the findings of the critical discourse analysis *situated within
aspects of the broader context* in which the discourses are produced,
circulated, and negotiated?

8   Have the researchers engaged in *reflexivity*?

9   Do the *results go beyond mere 'commenting'* on texts? Is the critical
intent of the study articulated?

Application to occupational science

There have been significant calls to incorporate methodologies into occupational
science that enable researchers to enhance understanding of 'occupation as situated' in political, economic, cultural, gendered, and other types of social conditions (Frank, 2012; Laliberte Rudman & Huot, 2013). We have found that critical
discourse analysis provides a methodology that enables us to enhance understanding of how injustices and inequities with regard to occupation and possibilities
to engage in occupation are discursively shaped and perpetuated. Using critical
discourse analysis to deconstruct taken-for-granted ideas and knowledge regarding occupation provides a means to enhance awareness of the social relations of
power that shape occupational possibilities in ways that privilege some groups
while simultaneously disadvantaging others. Such work can advance understanding of how occupation is governed, negotiated, and enacted at societal, collective,
and individual levels and inform actions aimed at supporting occupational rights.

Critical discourse analysis also provides a means to build upon the large
body of qualitative research that has focused on understanding the meaning of

occupation in the lives of individuals. Rather than locating meaning purely within individuals, critical discourse analysis provides a means to attend to questions "concerning the broad cultural and the institutional contexts of meaning making and social order" (Holstein & Gubrium, 2011, p. 342). By situating the meaning given to occupation by individuals within the contexts in which they live, we can advance understanding of how contextual features are embedded within how people view, and actively negotiate, themselves and their occupations.

Application to occupational therapy

Critical discourse analysis offers a promising methodology to understand how occupational therapy practice and professional knowledge is shaped within broader sociopolitical, as well as institutional, frames. Such research is important as occupational therapy practice is not only shaped by broader discourses but actively and constantly shapes itself and its assumptions, relations, and contexts through the discourses it produces and enacts. In their critical discourse analysis work addressing falling in older people and related health care practices, Ballinger and Payne (2000a) raised critical questions related to how the predominant use of biomedical discourses of health and illness and "a focus on falling may be at odds with the profession's self-proclaimed 'holistic' practices as occupational therapists" (p. 568). Understanding how specific discourses shape professional practice, in turn, can create possibilities for alternative viewpoints, changing practices, and resisting dominant discourses that constrain occupational therapy and other forms of health care practice (Ceci & Purkis, 2009; Lupton, 1992).

Authors' reflections

Our introductions to critical discourse analysis occurred within our doctoral dissertations. Finding that our view on the topics we were interested in – 'positive' aging and risk – were commensurate with a critical paradigm, critical discourse analysis, informed by a governmentality frame, enabled us to address questions regarding the sociopolitical shaping of occupational possibilities in relation to these topics. It is clear to us that critical discourse analysis would not fit well for researchers who are looking for a research approach that meticulously outlines what should be done and how it should be done, as critical discourse analysis demands engaging in a systematic, on-going process of ensuring a congruence between paradigm, theory, methodology, and methods. For Debbie, this methodology was particularly attractive as it provided a means for her to 'dig under' the assumptions that she had begun to question within her daily life and in her clinical work as an occupational therapist, regarding what it means to age and what occupations are appropriate, and inappropriate, for people as they age. For Silke, it was her interest in risk, its connection to power, and how risk discourses shape possibilities to engage in occupation that led her to critical discourse analysis. Working as an occupational therapist she encountered how concerns about 'safety' were able to justify or deny almost any change in work practice and became concerned regarding how fears of accountability seemed to be able to overrule individual needs and wishes, such as living independently. Within this reflection section, we highlight two additional challenges: (1) the 'unsettling' effect of questioning dominant ways of understanding a phenomenon and (2) the difficulty of stepping outside of and/or resisting being drawn into the discourses one is attempting to de-construct.

In questioning particular discourses, one begins to see that one's work is also a discursive production. Various types of knowledge one takes for granted and acts upon, in unnoticed ways, are also discursively produced. This might not only unsettle one's certainty in knowledge one has long drawn upon in one's professional, and perhaps personal, life but can also have a paralyzing effect in that one might fear to construct anything – given that any text produced itself is a discourse. For example, in de-constructing discourses of 'positive' aging that increasingly inform various types of health care practices, Debbie struggled with de-constructing aspects of such discourses that align with the value she, and occupational therapy, places on active engagement in occupations as a means to health. Debbie was also concerned that any alternative ways of writing and thinking about aging she produced within her own texts might inadvertently perpetuate aspects of positive aging discourses she had critiqued as marginalizing and exclusionary. It is our stance that in doing critical discourse analysis one needs to come to terms with operating within an ontological stance in which that which is taken as 'real' (including the knowledge created through one's analysis) is viewed as constructed and 'tentative' (Ainsworth & Hardy, 2004a). While this does not enable claims of 'scientific' certainty, it creates a sense of freedom as what is taken-for-granted is now seen as always changeable.

Further, critical discourse analysis is not about proving a discourse 'wrong', 'right', or replacing it with a 'better' one, as all discourses are constructions tied to particular viewpoints, values, and aims. We have both found it challenging, at times, to avoid being drawn into the discourses we are analyzing. For instance, when Silke, at the very beginning of the analysis noticed inconsistencies within what was presented as objective, scientifically derived 'facts' regarding aging drivers, she felt compelled to carve out the inconsistencies and faults of logic within them. Silke had been drawn into the powerful logic of the texts, endeavoring to replace one 'truth' with another 'truth', struck by the authorative ways texts provided information. Engaging in reflexivity, taking a step back and referring to her theoretical framework allowed Silke to shift analysis back to the effects of these constructed 'truths', that is, to focus on *how* particular facts about driving in later life become constructed as a given 'truth' and what power effects and constraints on occupational possibilities these constructions have. Stepping outside the logic of discourses which are part of the taken-for-granted reality in which our lives are lived is a related challenge – for example, it is difficult to question a construction of aging drivers as inherently increasingly risky in their driving or to question the promotion of continued engagement in volunteer work as a means to age well. In our work, this is where we both realize the importance of using a theoretical framework to guide all aspects of critical discourse analysis – using a governmentality framework provided us with a means to question such constructions, push beyond their apparent truthfulness, and focus on their power effects.

Summary

Critical discourse analysis demands that researchers take a stance and articulate the values and ideas that guide their analysis. Given the long-standing predominance of objectivist or positivist models of science within and outside of the occupation-based literature, choosing to do critical discourse analysis can be challenging. Indeed, Cheek (2004) has argued that critical discourse analysis exists at the margins of qualitative research, contending that this marginal position fruitfully allows critical discourse analysis to be used to transform understandings and question health care practices. We contend that critical discourse analysis studies can make vital contributions to advancing understandings of occupation and can be used to question and extend practices of both occupational scientists and occupational therapists. In order for this to occur, it is imperative that researchers who take up this methodology ensure that their theoretical underpinnings are commensurate with a critical paradigmatic view of language and discourse as social practice and that their research purposes encompass a critical intent.

References

Ainsworth, S., & Hardy, C. (2004a). Critical discourse analysis and identity: Why bother? *Critical Discourse Studies, 1*(2), 225–259. doi:10.1080/1740590042000302085.

Ainsworth, S., & Hardy, C. (2004b). Discourse and identities. In D. Grant, H. C. Oswick, & L. Putnam (Eds.), *The Sage handbook of organizational discourse analysis* (pp. 153–174). Thousand Oaks, CA: Sage.

Allen, D., & Hardin, P. K. (2001). Discourse analysis and the epidemiology of meaning. *Nursing Philosophy, 2*(2), 163–176. doi:10.1046/j.1466–769X.2001.00049.x.

Ballinger, C. (2006). Demonstrating rigour and quality? In L. Finlay & C. Ballinger (Eds.), *Qualitative research for allied health professionals: Challenging choices* (pp. 235–246). West Sussex, UK: John Wiley & Sons.

Ballinger, C., & Cheek, J. (2006). Discourse analysis in action: The construction of risk in a community day hospital. In L. Finlay & C. Ballinger (Eds.), *Qualitative research for allied health professionals: Challenging choices* (pp. 200–217). Chichester, UK: John Wiley & Sons.

Ballinger, C., & Payne, S. (2000a). Discourse analysis: Principles, applications and critique. *British Journal of Occupational Therapy, 63*(12), 566–572.

Ballinger, C., & Payne, S. (2000b). Falling from grace or into expert hands? Alternative accounts about falling in older people. *British Journal of Occupational Therapy, 63*(12), 573–579.

Ballinger, C., & Payne, S. (2002). The construction of risk of falling among and by older people. *Ageing and Society, 22*(2), 305–324. doi:10.1017/S0144686X02008620.

Castel, R. (1991). From dangerousness to risk. In G. Burchell, C. Gordon, & P. Miller (Eds.), *The Foucault effect: Studies in governmentality* (pp. 281–298). Chicago: University of Chicago Press.

Ceci, C., & Purkis, M. (2009). Bridging gaps in risk discourse: Home care case management and client choices. *Sociology of Health and Illness, 31*(2), 201–214. doi:10.1111/j.1467-9566.2008.01127.x.

Cheek, J. (2000). *Postmodern and poststructural approaches to nursing research.* Thousand Oaks, CA: Sage.

Cheek, J. (2004). At the margins? Discourse analysis and qualitative research. *Qualitative Health Research, 14*(8), 1140–1150. doi:10.1177/1049732304266820.

Crowe, M. (2001). Constructing normality: A discourse analysis of the DSM-IV. *Journal of Psychiatric and Mental Health Nursing, 7*(1), 69–77. doi:10.1046/j.1365–2850.2000. 00261.x.

Dennhardt, S. (2013). *Governing occupation through constructions of risk: The case of the aging driver.* Unpublished doctoral thesis. The University of Western Ontario, London, Ontario, Canada.

Dennhardt S., & Laliberte Rudman, D. (2012). When occupation goes 'wrong': A critical reflection on risk discourses and their relevance in shaping occupation. In G. E. Whiteford & C. Hocking (Eds.), *Occupational science: Society, inclusion and participation* (pp. 117–136). Oxford, UK: Wiley-Blackwell.

Fairclough, N. (1995). *Critical discourse analysis: The critical study of language.* London, UK: Longman.

Fairclough, N. (2009). A dialectical-relational approach to critical discourse analysis in social research. In R. Wodak & M. Meyer (Eds.), *Methods of critical discourse analysis* (2nd ed., pp. 162–186). Thousand Oaks, CA: Sage.

Foucault, M. (1972). *The archaeology of knowledge.* New York, NY: Pantheon.

Frank, G. (2012). The 2010 Ruth Zemke lecture in occupational science. Occupational therapy/occupational science/occupational justice: Moral commitments and global assemblages. *Journal of Occupational Science, 19*(1), 25–35. doi:10.1080/14427591. 2011.607792.

Hardin, P. K. (2001). Theory and language: Locating agency between free will and discursive marionettes. *Nursing Inquiry, 8*(1), 11–18. doi:10.1046/j.1440-1800.2001.00084.x.

Hardin, P. K. (2003). Constructing experience in individual interviews, autobiographies and on-line accounts: A poststructuralist approach. *Journal of Advancing Nursing, 41*(6), 536–544. doi:10.1046/j.1365-2648.2003.02565.x.

Hardy, C., & Phillips, N. (1999). No joking matter: Discursive struggle in the Canadian refugee system. *Organization Studies, 20*(1), 1–24. doi:10.1177/0170840699201001.

Hardy, C., & Phillips, N. (2004). Discourse and power. In D. Grant, C. Hardy, C. Oswick, & L. Putnam (Eds.), *The Sage handbook of organizational discourse* (pp. 299–316). Thousand Oaks, CA: Sage.

Holstein, J. A., & Gubrium, J. F. (2011). The constructionist analytics of interpretive practice. In N. K. Denzin & Y. S. Lincoln (Eds.), *The Sage handbook of qualitative research* (pp. 341–357). Thousand Oaks, CA: Sage.

Jäger, S., & Maier, F. (2009). Theoretical and methodological aspects of Foucauldian critical discourse analysis and dispositive analysis. In R. Wodak & M. Meyer (Eds.), *Methods of critical discourse analysis* (2nd ed., pp. 34–61). London, UK: Sage.

Johansson, K., Lilja, M., Park, M., & Josephsson, S. (2010). Balancing the good–a critical discourse analysis of home modification services. *Sociology of Health & Illness, 32*(4), 563–582. doi:10.1111/j.1467–9566.2009.01232.x.

Jørgensen, M., & Phillips, L. J. (2002). *Discourse analysis as theory and method.* London, UK: Sage.

Kantartzis, S., & Molineux, M. (2012). Understanding the discursive development of occupation: Historico-political perspectives. In G. E. Whiteford & C. Hocking (Eds.), *Occupational science: Society, inclusion, participation* (pp. 38–53). West Sussex, UK: Blackwell Publishing.

Laliberte Rudman, D. (2005). Understanding political influences on occupational possibilities: An analysis of newspaper constructions of retirees. *Journal of Occupational Science, 12*(3), 149–160. doi:10.1080/14427591.2005.9686558.

Laliberte Rudman, D. (2006). Shaping the active, autonomous and responsible modern retiree: An analysis of discursive technologies and their connections with neoliberal political rationality. *Ageing and Society, 26*, 181–201. doi:10.1017/S0144686X05004253.

Laliberte Rudman, D. (2010). Occupational possibilities. *Journal of Occupational Science, 17*(1), 55–59. doi:10.1080/14427591.2010.9686673.

Laliberte Rudman, D. (2013). Enacting the critical potential of occupational science: Problematizing the 'individualizing of occupation'. *Journal of Occupational Science, 20*(4), 298–313. doi:10.1080/14427591.2013.803434.

Laliberte Rudman, D. (2014). Reflecting on the socially situated and constructed nature of occupation: A research program addressing the contemporary restructuring of retirement. In D. Pierce (Ed.), *Occupational science for occupational therapy* (pp. 143–156). Thorofare, NJ: Slack.

Laliberte Rudman, D., & Huot, S. (2013). Conceptual insights for expanding thinking regarding the situated nature of occupation. In M. P. Cutchin & V. A. Dickie (Eds.), *Transactional perspectives on occupation* (pp. 51–64). New York, NY: Springer.

Laliberte Rudman, D., Huot, S., & Dennhardt, S. (2009). Shaping ideal places for retirement: Occupational possibilities within contemporary media. *Journal of Occupational Science, 16*(1), 18–24. doi:10.1080/14427591.2009.9686637.

Laliberte Rudman, D., & Molke, D. (2009). Forever productive: The discursive shaping of later life workers in contemporary Canadian newspapers. *WORK: A Journal of Prevention, Assessment & Rehabilitation, 32*(4), 377–390. doi:10.3233/WOR-2009-0850.

Lupton, D. (1992). Discourse analysis: A new methodology for understanding the ideologies of health and illness. *Australian Journal of Public Health, 16*(2), 145–150. doi:10.1111/j.1753-6405.1992.tb00043.x.

Millington, B. (2011). Use it or lose it: Ageing and the politics of brain training. *Leisure Studies, 31*(4), 429–446. doi:10.1080/02614367.2011.589865.

Mumby, D. K. (2004). Discourse, power and ideology: Unpacking the critical approach. In D. Grant, H. C. Oswick, & L. Putnam (Eds.), *The Sage handbook of organizational discourse analysis* (pp. 217–259). Thousand Oaks, CA: Sage.

Pereira, R. B. (2013). Using critical policy analysis in occupational science research: Exploring Bacchi's methodology. *Journal of Occupational Science.* doi:10.1080/144 27591.2013.806207.

Phillips, N., & Hardy, C. (2002). *Discourse analysis: Investigating processes of social construction.* Thousand Oaks, CA: Sage.

Richardson, J. E. (2007). *Analysing newspapers: An approach from critical discourse analysis.* New York, NY: Palgrave Macmillan.

Rose, G. (2007). *Visual methodologies: An introduction to the interpretation of visual materials* (2nd ed.). Thousand Oaks, CA: Sage.

van Dijk, T. A. (1997). Editorial: Analysing discourse analysis. *Discourse & Society, 8*(1), 5–6. doi:10.1177/0957926597008001001.

van Dijk, T. A. (2009). Critical discourse studies: A sociolinguistic approach. In R. Wodak & M. Meyer (Eds.), *Methods of critical discourse analysis* (2nd ed., pp. 62–86). Thousand Oaks, CA: Sage.

van Leeuwen, T. (2008). Representing social actors with toys. In T. van Leeuwen (Ed.), *Discourse and practice: New tools for critical discourse analysis* (pp. 149–162). Oxford, UK: Oxford University Press.

Wodak, R., & Meyer, M. (2009). Critical discourse analysis: History, agenda, theory and methodology. In R. Wodak & M. Meyer (Eds.), *Methods of critical discourse analysis* (2nd ed., pp. 1–33). Thousand Oaks, CA: Sage.

Wood, L. A., & Kroger, R. O. (2000). *Doing discourse analysis: Methods for studying action in talk and text*. Thousand Oaks, CA: Sage.

Further reading

Fairclough, N., & Wodak, R. (1997). Critical discourse analysis. In T. A. Van Dijk (Ed.), *Discourse as social interaction. Discourse studies: A multidisciplinary introduction* (pp. 258–284). Thousand Oaks, CA: Sage.

Grant, D., Hardy, C., Oswick, C., & Putnam, L. (Eds.). (2004). *The Sage handbook of organizational discourse*. Thousand Oaks, CA: Sage.

Kendall, G., & Wickham, G. (1999). *Using Foucault's methods*. London, UK: Sage.

Parker, I., & Bolton Discourse Network. (1999). *Critical textwork: An introduction to varieties of discourse and analysis*. Buckingham, UK: Open University Press.

Wodak, R., & Meyer, M. (2009). *Methods of critical discourse analysis* (2nd ed.). London, UK: Sage.

11 Visual methodologies

Photovoice in focus

Eric Asaba, Debbie Laliberte Rudman,
Margarita Mondaca, and Melissa Park

Visual images evoke elements of human consciousness that words alone cannot; images evoke both more information and different kinds of information (Harper, 2002). Not surprisingly, images are being utilized in research to access meaning. Visual research methods can be broadly defined as encompassing systematic ways in which visual materials are gathered or generated and worked with to understand, explain, or express phenomena – a process that is in constant development (Pink, 2012). For example, research can draw upon pre-existing photos or videos; alternatively photos and videos can be generated as a result of the research process. Moreover, visual materials can be generated by researchers, informants, or in collaboration (Prosser & Schwartz, 1998). Visual methods can be used for varying purposes such as documenting observations, capturing processes as they occur, or for facilitating dialog (Prosser, 2011; Prosser, Clark, & Wiles, 2008; Wang & Burris, 1997). The number of approaches to, and terminology for, visual methods has developed over the years to include photo elicitation, photo tour, video diaries, photo story, body mapping, film elicitation, photo novella, and photovoice. All these terms can be taken to reflect a set of assumptions about visual literacy – that visual artifacts can be "read" as a text (Catalani & Minkler, 2009; Elkins, 2008; Hartman, Mandich, Magalhaes, & Orchard, 2011; Lal, Jarus, & Suto, 2012; van Nes, Jonsson, Hirschier, Abma, & Deeg, 2012). James Elkins (2008), an art historian, wrote in his introduction to *Visual Literacy:*

> Since the 1980s the rhetoric of images has become far more pervasive, so that it is now commonplace in the media to hear that we live in a visual culture, and get our information through images. It is time, I think, to take those claims seriously. (p. 4)

Yet, although the possibilities for using visual materials are plentiful, a sense of caution must be exercised about assumptions around literacy or, more fundamentally, the notion of visual literacy in and of itself in this context. Elkins argued that scholars too often assume a certain literacy of visual images; this literacy needs to be learned. We suggest that reflecting upon how our epistemologies, or ways of knowing, in large part shape or determine how we "read" images and thus, suggest explicitly how reflecting on our epistemologies can focus our process of inquiry.

Much like the aperture on a camera, epistemologies focus what is foregrounded and what becomes part of the background. Visual images can serve as a tool to facilitate dialog in order to empower access or enrich understanding of experiences (Wang & Burris, 1994; Wang, Burris, & Ping, 1996), or as a symbolic representation of political or historical situations to stimulate dialog in the public realm for education, debate and/or policy changes (Carlson, Engebretson, & Chamberlain, 2006). All the authors of this chapter have utilized a variety of visual methods (including the use of video and drawings in addition to photography), either in the projects from which we draw in this chapter or in other projects. We have been active in discussions that have shaped both our pragmatic and conceptual understanding of visual methods, photovoice, analysis, and writing in relation to the projects from which we draw on in this chapter.

In this chapter, we have chosen to focus on photovoice, both because it allows us to draw from our experiences with projects that span three countries and because photovoice has appeared more and more in conference presentations within occupational science and occupational therapy. Conversely, literature within occupational science and occupational therapy in which photovoice is used only emerges after 2010 and is relatively sparse (Lal et al., 2012). We have found photovoice to be particularly useful in understanding questions related to occupation and its negotiation in everyday life and contend that the sense of immediacy and accessibility of visual images can provide a potent vehicle for knowledge mobilization, exchange, and transfer.

Vision Quests (Laliberte Rudman et al., 2010/2011) is a project which aimed to document Canadian First Nations youths' perspectives regarding the conditions that enable and limit their occupational transition to postsecondary education. The project Creating Inclusive Communities (Asaba et al., 2010) aimed to explore experiences among persons over the age of 60 who had undergone international migration; particularly focusing on what facilitates and/or hinders participation in local communities. Both projects utilized photovoice as a participatory methodology that involved a group of people producing, sharing, and discussing photos that pertain to shared experiences in order to enable people to (a) record and reflect strengths and barriers in their communities, (b) engage in critical dialog about important topics through group discussions of photographs, and (c) play an active role in reaching the public and policymakers. Members in a photovoice group capture essences of events or stories using photographs, which serve as a representation of daily sociopolitical realities experienced by the individual or group and function as a catalyst for further narrative exploration (Wang & Burris, 1994, 1997; Wang et al., 1996). Implicitly, we note how a participatory methodology in the Vision Quests project foregrounds the documentation of structural inequities and constraints, while a narrative methodology in the Creating Inclusive Communities foregrounds understanding experience.

Our ambition in this chapter is to use illustrations and reflections from these projects in order to provide initial guidance in planning, conducting, analyzing, and presenting photovoice research. Moreover, we will examine how epistemological orientations guided our choices in the field; specifically, how participatory and narrative approaches guided our approach to ethics, our relationships with those who were involved in our photovoice projects, and how data were generated. Although we will describe a process by which data can be generated and analyzed, we believe that the how-to steps have little value without understanding the 'what' and 'why' of the specific approach.

Background

Photovoice, initially referred to as photo novella, was coined by Wang and colleagues in a project focusing on maternal and child health in rural China (Wang & Burris, 1994, 1997; Wang et al., 1996). Wang et al. used photography as a method to engage a group of women who had experienced marginalization in order to impact on social change (Lal et al., 2012; Wang & Burris, 1997). Since then, photovoice has been widely applied within community-based research projects using a participatory methodology to empower groups who are viewed as marginalized within their local environment or who collectively desire to change aspects of their contexts, such as people with mental illness, people experiencing homelessness or poverty, people with severe physical disabilities, minorities, or older citizens (Castleden, Garvin, & Nation, 2008; Haque & Eng, 2011; Novek, Morris-Oswald, & Menec, 2012; Wang & Pies, 2008). Along with a common focus on groups who are viewed as marginalized or vulnerable, there is a commitment with photovoice to collectively identify barriers faced by such groups and bring to light the strengths, capacities, resources, and contributions of people.

Epistemology and positioning

Photovoice challenges the traditional power relation between *researchers* and *researched* (Carlson et al., 2006). Traditionally, researchers have been seen as possessing knowledge and have thus been in positions of power to make decisions about what and how to study given phenomena. In Creating Inclusive Communities (Asaba et al., 2010), following Sen (1992), a provision of resources or knowledge alone was seen as insufficient in impacting on social change; rather people needed to be able to convert resources into something personally meaningful and functional. This is conceptually important for three reasons.

First, participants in photovoice research projects are often people that are publicly considered to have access to fewer resources, yet their unique experiences can contribute to new knowledge and development of practices. Photovoice research advertently shifts focus from vulnerability as weakness to vulnerability as a common platform from which to actively pursue alternative possibilities. Second, photovoice research challenges the view of participant as a source of information and instead collaborates with participant as co-researcher in defining what information is of relevance given a general area of interest, generating possibilities to influence and reframe research inquiries. Third, photovoice can be a way to connect with community members (Carlson et al., 2006).

Just as the representational status of language has been questioned in narrative data (Garro & Mattingly, 2000; Riessman, 2008), epistemological questions about what visual data can represent and its socially constructed nature have been debated. Throughout the chapter, we raise epistemological questions that are more broadly applicable to thinking about how to approach the visual. For example, Harper (2002) discussed the various ways in which the social positions of the photographer and subject come into play when a photograph is taken and the need to consider who has the power to photograph. Once a shift is made away from a realist assumption that images 'speak' for themselves, there is greater demand on researchers to contextualize and interpret images (Prosser, 2011). We contend that it is particularly important to be reflexive regarding how the 'visual' is understood, constructed, and interpreted within any study (Banks, 2007; Prosser & Schwartz, 1998). Within photovoice, ideally, this act of interpretation is participatory; the people who generated the photos collectively discuss and interpret the photos in relation to the issues framing the project and the photo-taking. At the same time, we note, how the different methodologies and conceptual frameworks of the different projects discussed herein, as influenced by their underlying epistemologies, shaped how these projects developed over time (including interpretation/analysis).

Topics and research questions

The research question is often framed as having to do with addressing a knowledge gap, either in finding new knowledge or exploring new ways to understand phenomena. In photovoice, the research question ideally evolves out of collaboration with co-researchers (all participants in a project who are part of the social setting and/or group being studied). As such, research questions often reflect issues of relevance to a setting or group, and in this way contribute to defining the knowledge gap. In one of our photovoice groups, an example of a question originally posed was, "What characterizes possibilities and barriers to feeling included in society among older adults who have experienced international migration?" When we met participants in this project, they posed questions such as, "Why are we portrayed so poorly in media or why don't people see the resources we bring?" Further examples of research questions are provided in Table 11.1.

Table 11.1 Examples of research questions

Type	Example
Colloquial language	Why are we portrayed so poorly in media?
	Why don't people see the resources we bring?
Research language	What characterizes possibilities and barriers to feeling included in society among older adults who have experienced international migration?
	How can photographic techniques facilitate an understanding of sensory experiences?

From the perspective of being inclusive, photovoice can be useful in that it does not necessarily demand the ability to read or write and taps into modes of expression beyond talk (Wang & Pies, 2008). Prosser and Schwartz (1998) wrote as follows:

> Photographs may not provide us with unbiased, objective documentation of the social and material world, but they can show characteristics and attributes of people, objects and events that often elude even the most skilled wordsmiths. (p. 335)

Hence, one of the advantages of photovoice is its wide accessibility for participants whose perspectives might otherwise be excluded from research.

Methodology

There are three major theoretical influences on the development of photovoice. First, photovoice incorporates Paulo Freire's approach to critical education in that it emphasizes "people's sharing and speaking from their own experience" (Wang & Pies, 2008, p. 184), the need for people to identify "the historical and social patterns that bind their individual lives together" (Wang & Pies, 2008, p. 184), and the capacity of people to generate collective solutions for enacting change (Freire, 1970, 1973; Wang & Burris, 1994; Wang & Pies, 2008). Freire (1973) emphasized reflexive discussions of everyday problems within communities in order to evoke social transformation. Second, photovoice has also been influenced by critical feminist theory, emphasizing voice and a platform for vantage points expressed by those who have or are experiencing some form of oppression (Wang & Pies, 2008). Third, theoretical underpinnings commonly associated with documentary photography are seen as particularly relevant with regard to how the camera functions as a tool in a process of empowerment and capacity building (Castleden et al., 2008).

Photovoice groups generate and discuss photographs in a project in order to facilitate the identification and representation of problems in a local community (Wang & Burris, 1997). There is an underlying assumption that by producing visual images, participants can convey their particular experiences while the forum for dialog about the photos can raise critical awareness of social forces through a collaborative process (Wang & Pies, 2008). Thus, photovoice can be conceptualized as situated methodologically between narrative and participatory approaches (Chapters 6 and 8). Our lenses in this chapter illustrate how the focus in two different research projects (i.e., questions/description of projects), foregrounded or backgrounded the participatory or narrative approaches.

Recruitment

Wang and Burris (1997) asserted that "the ideal 'who' or 'where' for using photovoice is a community or group in which people are involved in all major phases of selecting and planning the process" (p. 377). A simple visual overview of phases from recruitment to exhibition based on our experiences is provided (Figure 11.1). In photovoice, recruitment is not about selecting a representative sample of people but rather about collaborating to define what parameters to apply in looking for partners (partnering). For instance, in the Vision Quests project, a mixture of personnel from local reserve communities whose positions address work and/or health, the Director of Indigenous Services at the local university, and a First Nations undergraduate student, among more, were invited to initial discussions for a project. Building upon an engaging process, potential research foci were discussed as well as ethical issues and principles of research outlined by both indigenous and research organizations in Canada to guide the conduct of research with indigenous peoples. Everyone was subsequently invited to be part of a grant proposal, thereby involved from the onset of planning the project that had a focus on youth in secondary education. Close collaboration in partnering in this way can be a merit if it is important the research design closely reflects the communities local knowledge, for instance the need to (a) include elders in the research process to ensure cultural safety and guidance for the youth; (b) provide a space for the youth to individually talk about their photos before bringing them to a group; (c) ensure youth had multiple decision points regarding what photos they would share and in what contexts; and (d) take a strengths-based approach, learning from and with youth who were succeeding in the transition (versus focusing on those who had dropped out).

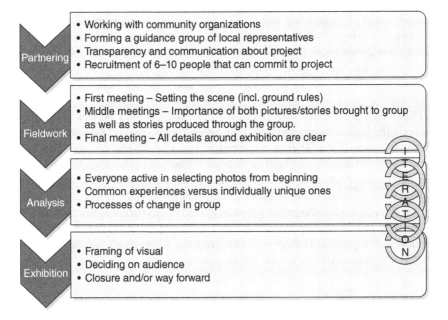

Figure 11.1 The photovoice process

Data gathering/data generation

Because of the nature in which photovoice groups work with data, we suggest that it can be useful to think in terms of generating data rather than gathering data. Although group sessions and discussions are often recorded using audio or video and later transcribed, in this way similar to many other qualitative data gathering methods, there is a collaborative idea about the generation of this data and in particular the pictures brought to sessions. Wang and Burris (1997) described the challenge of offering guidelines that open up possibilities and build on community strengths rather than using language and methodological structures that limit or "pathologize" (p. 378) people. This is important because the line between facilitating and leading a group is thin, and in the case of photovoice, a risk is that the facilitator's voice becomes too strong, thereby contributing negatively to ideals of empowerment and participation. The number of sessions held, the duration of data generation, or the number of members appropriate for a group all depend on the context and questions characterizing the project. We have found that less than 5 members can at times feel like too few, especially if someone is ill or needs to miss a meeting; conversely more than 10 members in a group can lead to limitations in time for each person to share. In the Creating Inclusive Communities project we found that 4 weeks was insufficient in establishing trust, planning, discussing, and finishing with a public exhibition or event where experiences are communicated to other stakeholders and community members. The precise instructions for running a photovoice group will thus vary greatly depending on circumstances. Here we put forth five reflections that can guide a process of planning data generation.

Lessons from the field 1: At the first meeting with a photovoice group, it can be relevant to describe the project and overall aims, do a round of introductions, discuss and establish ground rules for the group, as well as decide on times to meet. It is important that group members feel safe and that everyone can participate on equal terms. Although a photovoice group might be homogenous from a sociopolitical perspective such as being of ethnic minority, homeless, or a migrant worker, members of a group might see each other as diverse in terms of values and customs. For this reason, we have found it relevant to allocate time during the first session to let each person share about themselves and talk about ground rules. Ground rules can consist of things such as being on time, calling if late, and not answering a mobile telephone during group time. It is important the group jointly agrees on the processes. Deciding on a time frame and schedule allows everyone to commit to and plan their presence and participation. We have found this structure instrumental in ensuring continuity. However, it has also been important to remain flexible to changes proposed by the group. For instance, in one of our projects, the group initially agreed to only meet for 2 hours per week during an 8-week period. However, at the second session participants communicated that 2 hours was not enough time and subsequent sessions were extended to 3 hours. At week 6, participants agreed that more time was needed to complete their work, thus the duration for the group was extended another 4 weeks with a holiday break in between. In this way, the group decided the amount of time spent conducting group work. Certain cultural rituals were also acknowledged, for example 'fika' in Sweden (Swedish custom of sharing coffee/tea and something to eat between a day's main meals).

Lessons from the field 2: To instruct in the use of a camera, or not? In most cases it is reasonable to provide basic instruction on how to use the provided camera, assuming that each participant is not using their own camera with which they are already familiar. By basic instruction we mean ensuring that everyone knows how to turn the camera on/off (digital), press the shutter (digital or analog), wind the camera (analog), delete an undesired picture (digital), and change batteries (digital). Where opinions diverge is the degree to which facilitators/researchers should provide instruction in *how* to take a picture. On the one hand, esthetically pleasing photographs with particular attention to focus, framing, depth, or color can be desirable; conversely, a focus on such elements can be detrimental to the metaphoric qualities or in-the-moment experiences of the photographer. If much time is spent on how-to instruction pertaining to photography, people are likely to produce photographs in keeping with a style in which they received instruction. Focusing on how-to can also lead to feeling pressured to produce a particular type of picture or a certain quality, which at times can stifle creativity or a freedom to express something that is not yet well understood for oneself. By not providing instruction, people are less likely to be steered in a particular direction with regard to how to take a picture; however, there can be frustration with feeling a lack of skill or later feeling that a picture does not esthetically measure up to a desired quality for an exhibition. These latter concerns can be dealt with more readily in a photovoice project through discussion and group processes as well as captions or written texts during exhibitions.

Lessons from the field 3: Groupwork with pictures. In most photovoice projects, sharing stories about pictures with others in a group serves as an important part of generating data. Castleden et al. (2008), in working with First Nations youth, raised concerns regarding the risks of participation in focus groups as well as the cultural appropriateness. Similarly, community partners in the Vision Quests project raised concerns regarding the discomfort that a group session might evoke for the youth, suggesting that it was important for the youth to have an opportunity to share and discuss their photos on a one-to-one basis with another First Nations youth. In addition, community partners, and elders, expressed that once such interviews were done, group sessions paralleled traditional 'Sharing Circles', in which each person is given space to talk if they so choose, would be an effective way for youth to share their thoughts and experiences with each other. Thus, generating data can vary broadly between projects depending on the aim, research question, and community need.

Lessons from the field 4: Frequency of meetings. A benefit of not meeting frequently is that there is much room for freedom in scheduling and requires less time from already busy lives. On the other hand, the continuity of meeting and sharing on a regular basis can provide a sense of belonging and the possibility to change direction in relation to emerging topics. Whatever the interval of gathering visual material, an important aspect of photovoice research is that members have an opportunity to explore what the picture represents for each person and what the picture can communicate about the individual as well as shared experiences.

Lessons from the field 5: Participatory processes with extensive photographic material. The longer a project runs, the more pictures are likely to be produced. In this sense, it is also relevant to consider how pictures are stored. A systematic way of storing and retrieving pictures will be particularly helpful when planning the final exhibition. In one of our projects where we had more than 700 photos, the group decided that each member/photographer would choose three pictures from each session that he or she wanted to put in an archive. By doing this, the group was able to begin with approximately 80 pictures instead of 700 when discussing which pictures to include and how to frame the exhibition.

Analysis

In photovoice research, the analysis begins when group members commence sharing ideas about the meanings of pictures. The sharing of pictures is therefore not merely an event of viewing the "gathered data" but rather a collaborative event of sharing experiences and beginning to interpret the visual and experiential information.

> Photovoice is not intended to produce a body of visual data for exhaustive analysis in the social science sense. . . . In contrast, photovoice offers a new framework and paradigm in which participants drive the analysis – from selecting photographs that they feel are most important or simply like best to the 'decoding' or descriptive interpretation of the images. (Wang & Pies, 2008, p. 192)

The methodological plasticity of photovoice means that participants can shape and tailor both the information gathered as well as the way in which this information is analyzed. This is important because in cases where participants in a project have experienced social exclusion or alienation from participation in local activities, it is likely that new ideas come up spontaneously during group work. For example, in the Vision Quests project, a participant presented photographs in a storied form, which influenced the group to adopt a photo-narrative approach to presenting stories through pictures. This provided a presentation of experiences across time and context as well as thematically presenting common experiences among participants. In this way, analysis was performed through group discussions and engagement in a process of writing detailed descriptions relating to concrete or symbolic aspects of each photo (Van Leeuwen, 2001).

It is also possible that certain experiences of relevance that have been dormant can come to be expressed because of the empowerment felt through a group where several people share similar experiences. For example, in one of our projects a member brought a picture of a dandelion, which had been taken during late autumn when dandelions typically are not in bloom (Figure 11.2). For the person

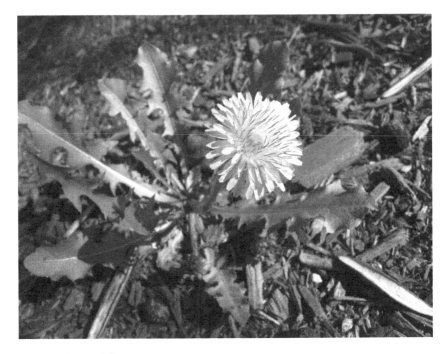

Figure 11.2 Dandelion

who took the photograph, the dandelion first represented beauty and strength in later life, the ability to bloom even during late autumn days, but through the group's discussion it also came to represent national policies around immigration (dandelion as weed or as the metaphorical burden in a garden) and the inevitable fact of modern migration (even if the dandelion is weeded it will keep returning, metaphorically migration will continue to occur even in light of barriers and challenges).

Dissemination

Another important dimension of the analytic process in photovoice is the reflexive and collaborative work of deciding how to present visual material in a way that communicates experiences aligned with the group's process and the objectives of the project. In the project in which the picture of the dandelion was taken, an artist was invited to discuss framing and displaying the photographs. The artist joined the group on two occasions. The first time she listened to participant stories, what they wanted to express, and the types of spaces in which the pictures would be displayed. She then provided concrete examples and feedback to the group about alternatives for the visual presentation of the pictures depending on color schemes, size, framing, height from ground, and symmetry versus asymmetry, among more. The second time the artist took part in the emerging display of photographs and discussion, again providing feedback. This time the feedback was given as a reflection about how the artist interpreted the presentation in order for the group to make decisions about whether this was what the group in fact intended or wished to express. Whether this level of work with esthetics is required or whether it is positive can be contended. Not every project in which we have worked has devoted this amount of time and detail to issues of presentation. We have found the contribution of an artist of value in making expressions more clear and in raising a sense of pride in the group's work. This was also not something that was planned rather something that grew from the group processes.

The outcome of analyses in a photovoice project can vary. In most cases the outcome is at least a photographic exhibition where a community/audience is invited to the visual (and often textual via captions) expression of experiences as well as a dialog with the group. Achieving social change or impacting directly on the community in which the project is conducted is a central tenet in photovoice. However, it should also be noted that the measure of social change is a debated concept. In many cases, researchers involved in a project also have academic career interests or grant obligations where scientific publication is an outcome. Authorship and co-authorship here can be negotiated as in any group where a joint work is produced. Thus, the analysis from photovoice can be in the form of a live or virtual visual exhibition where photos have been selected for a particular illustration (Figure 11.3), an open lecture in storied form accompanying photographs, or a thematic analysis of shared experiences. Moreover, these analyses can be presented at a community center or in a scientific publication where theory and other relevant methods are drawn upon. It is rare that pictures are analyzed for content, since photographs are used as catalysts for discussion and are used as representations for something that someone in a group wants to highlight.

Ethics and rigor

Ethical aspects of conducting photovoice research are of critical importance. This section has both an instrumental aspect related to informed consent and the use of visual material, as well as a reflective aspect related to challenges we have come across in conducting our projects.

Photovoice entails certain additional ethical challenges as compared to other qualitative or participatory methods because photos are used (Wang & Redwood-Jones, 2001); for example, the act of taking pictures in a community is a political act that both discloses that which is photographed and hides what is not. Photography can be intrusive and lead to unintended consequences (Castleden et al., 2008). Dealing with anonymity and confidentiality is also challenging, although strategies such as addressing ethics in photovoice training sessions, using informed consent forms (from those photographed), transcription verification (allowing participants to delete any potentially harmful photos and transcripts), and photo release forms (ensure understanding of what photos would be used for and where photographs would be published) are used. Photovoice projects often involve people who

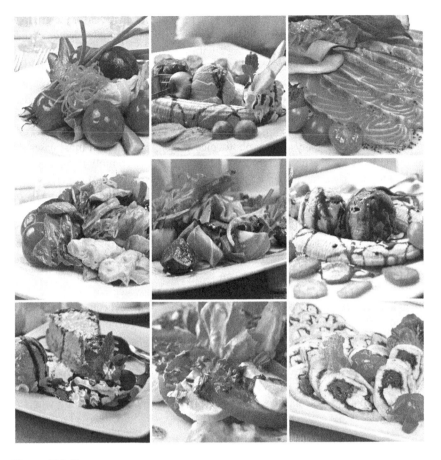

Figure 11.3 Sensory

are 'vulnerable'/marginalized; it is thus critical to emphasize that no picture is worth taking if it brings the photographer or subject of the photograph harm (see Table 11.2 for potential risks).

Photovoice research projects need to be anchored in a local context and in struggles experienced by the participants, otherwise there is a risk of it being used as an instrumental approach to gathering photos as a complement to group interviews. If there is a lack of participatory elements that are central within an epistemology of photovoice research, then projects that do not involve group discussion, stakeholder consultation, or identification of action strategies do not meet the rigor of being participatory. Lal et al. (2012) argued that sole reliance on individual interviews regarding photos, as opposed to group discussions, significantly detracts from the positive effects that arise from enactment of participatory principles and a transformative group context. It has been argued that if the

Table 11.2 Potential risks and strategies for working with risks

Potential risks	Strategies
Taking pictures that portray community, group, or individuals in a negative light	Discussing risks and ensuring match between member resources and aim of project
Pointing out a group/community as 'marginalized', 'oppressed', and 'vulnerable'. Can contribute to stigmatization and further marginalization of group	Being attentive to language use, discussion around risks associated with presentations, and having representative reference groups
Photography can be interpreted as intrusive	Discussion about informed consent and forms needed when taking pictures of people
People in pictures are no longer anonymous	Discussion of informed consent and possible risks of being identified in a photo
Excluding people who might be seen as limited in taking pictures due to physical, sensory, or cognitive barriers – consider how techniques can be adapted	Working with reference groups to find adaptive strategies to make project inclusive

methodology does not contain an action component where photos and discussions do not come from community members, then it should not be labeled as photovoice (Hartman et al., 2011).

Another aspect is the need for redefinition of power positions and relationships; experts are the participants themselves, whereas researchers are often acknowledged as resources that can facilitate the negotiated and sanctioned agendas pertaining to the identified social issues. A perpetual challenge in photovoice projects is future sustainability of social actions in line with the social issues identified by the group. Researchers and participants might create collaborations with organized local partners and multiple social actors as part of a network that aims to continue when formal research processes have been concluded.

There are limits to what is observable and what can be photographed – both for practical and ethical reasons (Castleden et al., 2008); while we found participants to be incredibly creative in how they used photos to comment on nontangible items or issues, we also found that combining photos with individual interviews opened up space for discussion regarding the issues that participants could not photograph. For example, in the Vision Quests project, racism emerged as an issue in the transition to and staying in post-secondary education. Visually representing racism as personally experienced in contemporary contexts was a challenge – most photos often referred to racism as experienced by others. However, in follow-up interviews, these photos often lead to discussion of personal experiences of racism. For example, one youth took photos of various historical artifacts

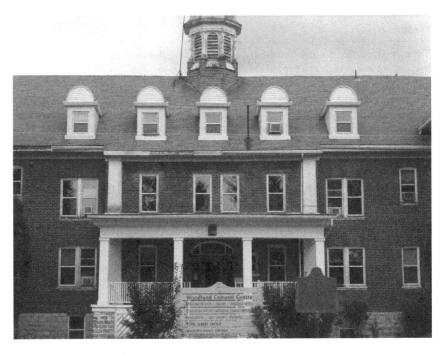

Figure 11.4 Residential school

regarding colonial practices used to assimilate and subjugate First Nations people (Figures 11.4 and 11.5). Within her interview, this youth expanded on her visual images of historical racist practices to explicate her own experiences of being stereotyped and having her capabilities being underestimated by teachers and peers.

The democratic ideal of an equal partnership emphasizes the unique strengths, expertise, and shared responsibility of all partners who are engaged in a joint process and involves all partners' input into all phases of a project. However, achieving equal participation and power can be challenging for various reasons; for example, in one project, two of the executive directors who were part of the project group left their organizational positions in the latter phases of the project, and the project focus was negotiated with the mandate of a funding source. Three partnering organizations wanted to have input in shaping the research questions and being part of community presentation of findings where potential action strategies were discussed, but at the same time indicated they did not have time or interest to participate in the photovoice process or in analysis. This raises questions about what counts as 'participatory'. Similarly, participants in another one of our projects expressed that they did not want to spend time in the latter parts of the analytic process through creating an exhibition. Rather they suggested that the researchers could make a suggestion to which they could make revisions. Cargo and Mercer (2008) have raised a distinction between equal and equitable

CANADA

DEPARTMENT OF INDIAN AFFAIRS

CIRCULAR   OTTAWA, 15th December, 1921.

Sir,-

It is observed with alarm that the holding of dances by the Indians on their reserves is on the increase, and that these practices tend to disorganize the efforts which the Department is putting forth to make them self-supporting.

I have, therefore, to direct you to use your utmost endeavours to dissuade the Indians from excessive indulgence in the practice of dancing. You should suppress any dances which cause waste of time, interfere with the occupations of the Indians, unsettle them for serious work, injure their health or encourage them in sloth and idleness. You should also dissuade, and, if possible, prevent them from leaving their reserves for the purpose of attending fairs, exhibitions, etc., when their absence would result in their own farming and other interests being neglected. It is realized that reasonable amusement and recreation should be enjoyed by Indians, but they should not be allowed to dissipate their energies and abandon themselves to demoralizing amusements. By the use of tact and firmness you can obtain control and keep it, and this obstacle to continued progress will then disappear.

The rooms, halls or other places in which Indians congregate should be under constant inspection. They should be scrubbed, fumigated, cleansed or disinfected to prevent the dissemination of disease. The Indians should be instructed in regard to the matter of proper ventilation and the avoidance of over-crowding rooms where public assemblies are being held, and proper arrangement should be made for the shelter of their horses and ponies. The Agent will avail himself of the services of the medical attendant of his agency in this connection.

Except where further information is desired, there will be no necessity to acknowledge the receipt of this circular.

Yours very truly,

Duncan Scott

Deputy Superintendent General.

Thos. Graham, Esq.,
    Indian Agent,
        Brocket, Alta.

Figure 11.5 The Indian Act

partnership, which we find useful here; an equitable partnership enables the contribution of each partner to be negotiated, rather than expected, and to align with each partner's resources and strengths.

Finally, how to handle social interactions and dynamics between group members within the research processes can be challenging. One woman in one of our projects became very invested in the ideas of being part of the group and making a change. She consistently came with pictures that she had taken and expected a platform to share these ideas at length. At times this led to conflict. In retrospect, and after some reflection, it is also interesting to think about what it was that got this person so invested in the questions and the process. Her passion and commitment was in many ways an expression and affirmation of the "empowerment" upon which the method in part rests. Her part in the group also led to "conflicts" and "making up", which in part also led to discussion around issues that allowed for the group to reach deeper insights about "participation" and investment in a process. She was perhaps also the one person from our projects who explicitly expressed how she would integrate photovoice ideas in her lifestyle.

Critiquing photovoice studies

The following questions in Textbox 11.1 have been developed to guide readers in critiquing studies using a photovoice methodology.

Textbox 11.1 Critiquing photovoice studies – questions to ask

1   To what degree is the problem/challenge *grounded in a local context*?
2   To what degree is the *data generating process participatory*?
3   How does the interpretive process provide *space for collective discussion and analysis*?
4   How is *authorship* of the generated data addressed in the project?
5   Are the authors *transparent regarding how ethical guidelines* for photo taking and exhibition were established?
6   Is there a *resulting photo exhibition*? To what degree is it collaborative and who constitutes the audience?
7   *What are the epistemologies* underlying not only the research question but those that guide the various researchers' and participants' on the team?
8   How are *sustainability issues* addressed with the community/local context?
9   How is the project *transformative of the societal challenge* addressed?

Application to occupational science

Drawing on photovoice to examine barriers and constraints to occupational engagement for groups experiencing marginalization has potential to enhance understanding of the ways in which various layers and elements of contexts influence the occupations in which individuals and collectives engage. For instance, photovoice can be a useful approach in projects where occupational deprivation (Wilcock, 1993, 1998) is in focus and where locally rooted change is of interest. In keeping with Hartman et al. (2011), we found that photovoice can advance the study of occupation through enabling researchers to gain access to tacit and commonplace elements of occupation that individuals have difficulty verbally describing as in our studies. The use of visual methods can also bring to light cultural elements of occupation (Berinstein & Magalhaes, 2009), ways in which curriculums exclude indigenous ways of knowing and doing and thereby limit occupational possibilities (Laliberte Rudman et al., 2010/2011), or experiences of aging between places among international migrants (Asaba et al., 2010). Finally, photovoice is inherently occupational in the sense that engagement in the project essentially means that people will plan things, do things, reflect on their plans and engagements, share in other people's experiences, as well as communicate all this visually, textually, and/or verbally. We also advocate for reflecting on the epistemologies guiding the projects. Not only is this part of our shared task of articulating our epistemic communities (Kinsella, 2012) but it also foregrounds or backgrounds the degree of focus we maintain on the personal and/or political aspects of a project.

Application to occupational therapy

Besides our work, there are many examples of how photovoice has been used to involve communities in health promotion initiatives and to inform health policies, systems, and programs (Wang & Pies, 2008). Given that the focus on participation and collaboration aligns well with client-centered approaches in occupational therapy practice, as does the use of activity and group work (Lal et al., 2012), photovoice can be taken to inform both occupational therapy as well as broader health care practices relevant to occupation. Photovoice can be used to address many types of research aims relevant for informing occupational therapy practice and advocacy, such as raising awareness around environmental barriers to participation, engaging in a group process aimed at changing aspects of peoples' daily lives, or communicating experiences of marginalization to key stakeholder groups (Lal et al., 2012).

Personal reflections

In medical sciences, the term bench-to-bedside has been used to conceptualize the need for not only translating scientific discoveries from animals to humans, but also to the actual spaces and places where people are receiving healthcare. What intrigued us about photovoice was the ambition of collaborating with people in a process that would both contribute to building knowledge in an academic sense and have a direct impact on communities/organizations in which the work was being carried out. By using visual materials, in combination with individual and group work, the depth of understanding and richness of information gathered was an advantage in this type of a research process.

Conclusion

Photovoice research requires a comfort with the unknown, a readiness to embrace the unexpected, and the patience to let the group process unravel in organic ways. For occupational therapy practitioners, the theoretical underpinnings of photovoice and our examples drawn from two projects can be used to focus attention on how the methodology of photovoice aligns with underlying assumptions in the practice of occupational therapy; that is, how healing occurs through engagement in occupations and how the potential of visual images can support this transformation. For occupational scientists, we hope that a focus on epistemologies sheds light on implications for rigor in the continued development of the "science" of occupation.

References

Asaba, E., Laliberte-Rudman, D., Park, M., Borell, L., Kottorp, A., Josephsson, S., & Luborsky, M. (2010). *Creating inclusive communities: Challenging the status quo through a multi-national innovative integration of ethnography and photovoice among elder migrants.* The Toyota Foundation – (Grant #D10-R-0076).

Banks, M. (2007). *Using visual data in qualitative research.* London, UK: Sage.

Berinstein, S., & Magalhaes, L. (2009). A study of the essence of play experience to children living in Zanzibar, Tanzania. *Occupational Therapy International, 16*(2), 89–106.

Cargo, M., & Mercer, S. L. (2008). The value and challenges of participatory research: Strengthening its practice. *Annual Review of Public Health, 29*, 325–350.

Carlson, E. D., Engebretson, J., & Chamberlain, R. M. (2006). Photovoice as a social process of critical consciousness. *Qualitative Health Research, 16*(6), 836–852.

Castleden, H., Garvin, T., & Nation, H.-a.-a. F. (2008). Modifying photovoice for community-based participatory indigenous research. *Social Science & Medicine, 66*(6), 1393–1405.

Catalani, C., & Minkler, M. (2009). Photovoice: A review of the literature in health and public health. *Health Education and Behaviour, 73*(3), 424–451. doi:1090198109342084 [pii]10.1177/1090198109342084.

Elkins, J. (Ed.). (2008). *Visual literacy.* New York, NY: Routledge.

Freire, P. (1970). *Pedagogy of the oppressed.* New York, NY: Continuum International Publishing Group.

Freire, P. (1973). *Education for critical consciousness.* New York, NY: Continuum Publishing Company.

Garro, L. C., & Mattingly, C. (2000). Narrative as construct and construction. In C. Mattingly & L. C. Garro (Eds.), *Narrative and the cultural construction of illness and healing* (pp. 1–49). Berkeley, CA: University of California Press.

Haque, N., & Eng, B. (2011). Tackling inequity through a Photovoice project on the social determinants of health. Translating Photovoice evidence to community action. *Global Health Promotion, 18*(1), 16–19.

Harper, D. (2002). Talking about pictures: A case for photo elicitation. *Visual Studies, 17*(1), 12–36.

Hartman, L. R., Mandich, A., Magalhaes, L., & Orchard, T. (2011). How do we "see" occupations? An examination of visual research methodologies in the study of human occupation. *Journal of Occupational Science, 18*(4), 292–305. doi:10.1080/14427591.2011.610776.

Kinsella, E. A. (2012). Knowledge paradigms in occupational science: Pluralistic perspectives. In G. E. Whiteford & C. Hocking (Eds.), *Occupational science: Society, inclusion, participation* (pp. 69–85). Oxford, UK: Wiley-Blackwell.

Lal, S., Jarus, T., & Suto, M. J. (2012). A scoping review of the photovoice method: Implications for occuaptional therapy research. *Canadian Journal of Occupational Therapy, 79*(3), 181–190.

Laliberte Rudman, D., Richmond, C., Huot, S., Klinger, L., Maghalaes, L., Mandich, A., . . . White, J. (2010/2011). Learning with First Nations Youth: A Photovoice study addressing visions of education and work success (in partnerhsip with Indigenous Services at Western N'Amerind Friendship Centre and Southwestern Ontario Aboriginal Health Access Centre): Social Sciences and Humanities Research Council of Canada, Aboriginal Research Program, Development Grant.

Novek, S., Morris-Oswald, T., & Menec, V. (2012). Using photovoice with older adults: Some methodological strengths and issues. *Aging and Society, 32*(3), 451–470.

Pink, S. (Ed.). (2012). *Advances in visual methodology*. London, UK: Sage.

Prosser, J. (2011). Visual methodology: Toward a more seeing research. In N. K. Denzin & Y. S. Lincoln (Eds.), *The Sage handbook of qualitative research* (4th ed., pp. 479–496). Los Angeles, CA: Sage.

Prosser, J., Clark, A., & Wiles, R. (2008). *Visual research ethics at the crossroads.* Reality Working Paper 10: University of Manchester, UK: ESRC National Centre for Research Methods.

Prosser, J., & Schwartz, D. (1998). Photographs within the sociological research process. In J. Prosser (Ed.), *Image-based research: A sourcebook for qualitative researchers* (pp. 706–721). London, UK: Falmer Press.

Riessman, C. K. (2008). *Narrative methods for the human sciences.* Thousand Oaks, CA: Sage.

Sen, A. (1992). *Inequality reexamined.* Cambridge, MA: Harvard University Press.

Van Leeuwen, T. (2001). Semiotics and iconography. In T. Van Leeuwen & C. Jewitt (Eds.), *Handbook of Visual Analysis* (pp. 92–118). London, UK: Sage.

van Nes, F., Jonsson, H., Hirschier, S., Abma, T., & Deeg, D. (2012). Meanings created in co-occupation: Construction of a late-life couple's photo story. *Journal of Occupational Science, 19*(4), 341–357. doi:10.1080/14427591.2012.679604.

Wang, C., & Burris, M. A. (1994). Empowerment through photo novella: Portraits of participation. *Health Education Quarterly, 21*(2), 171–186.

Wang, C., & Burris, M. A. (1997). Photovoice: Concept, methodology, and use for participatory needs assessment. *Health Education Behaviour, 24*(3), 369–387.

Wang, C., Burris, M. A., & Ping, X. Y. (1996). Chinese village women as visual anthropologists: A participatory approach to reaching policymakers. *Social Science & Medicine, 42*(10), 1391–1400. doi: 0277953695002871.

Wang, C., & Pies. (2008). Local knowledge, local power, and collective action. In P. Liamputtong (Ed.), *Performing qualitative cross-cultural research* (pp. 186–211). Cambridge, UK: Cambridge University Press.

Wang, C., & Redwood-Jones, Y. A. (2001). Photovoice ethics: Perspectives from flint photovoice. *Health Education & Behavior, 28*(5), 560–572.

Wilcock, A. (1993). A theory of the human need for occupation. *Journal of Occupational Science, 1*(1), 17–24.

Wilcock, A. (1998). *An occupational perspective of health.* Thorofare, NJ: SLACK.

Websites

http://www.photovoice.org/
http://photovoice.ca/
http://www.photovoicesinternational.org/
http://photovoice-research.com/
Gastaldo, D., Magalhaes, L, Carrasco, C., & Davy, C. (2013). *Body-Map: Storytelling as research.* Creative Commons. http://www.migrationhealth.ca/undocumented-workers-ontario/body-mapping.

12 Meta-synthesis demystified
Connecting islands of knowledge

Carolyn Murray and Mandy Stanley

An oft heard critique of qualitative research is the size of the sample despite the richness of the data far outweighing considerations of sample size. Meta-synthesis offers an approach which can connect those small islands of knowledge generated in qualitative studies to build a greater whole. In this chapter, we outline the history and origins of the meta-synthesis approach, and some of the debates and tensions in the meta-synthesis literature. More importantly, however, we aim to demystify an approach which has growing utility for occupational scientists and occupational therapists and yet remains largely unknown and under-utilized. We aim to leave you with the idea that a meta-synthesis approach is something that may be within your skills, is achievable, worthwhile, and is not just for research experts. However, like any qualitative approach, it requires considerable effort – so be prepared to embrace ambiguity and take the time to be creative while concepts and ideas take shape (Paterson et al., 2009).

As authors of this chapter, we do not hold ourselves out to be experts in meta-synthesis; rather we consider ourselves as researchers who have had some experience and are prepared to share our struggles and learning. We are both experienced occupational therapy educators and identify with being qualitative researchers. Additionally, we both have experience with supervising Honors students doing qualitative work, and Mandy has supervised several doctoral students to successful completion. The opportunity to extend our repertoire of knowledge and skill in qualitative methodologies arose during Carolyn's honors project in 2012 when she decided to tackle a meta-synthesis. The learnings from that study (Murray, Stanley, & Wright, 2013), and others, inform this chapter.

Occupational scientists and occupational therapists are attracted to qualitative methodologies because of the philosophy of client-centeredness and an inherent interest in how others perceive the world (Frank & Polkinghorne, 2010; Tomlin & Borgetto, 2011). Thus, qualitative research studies in occupational science and occupational therapy characteristically have small sample sizes which provide rich in-depth explorations of experience and perspectives (Sandelowski, 2000). Despite being rich and insightful, qualitative studies with small sample sizes are likely to get excluded from systematic reviews and clinical guidelines because of the inherent epistemological difference from quantitative research nor do they have the numerical data for extraction into a meta-analysis (Taylor, 2007).

Notwithstanding the insights that qualitative research provides, the likelihood of translation into practice is low, and Pearson (2004, p. 61) proposed that it is time for evidence-based approaches to move beyond measuring 'effectiveness' of interventions to also consider "feasibility, appropriateness and meaningfulness" of consumer contact with practitioners. If the findings from smaller qualitative studies are brought together through development of consistent and rigorous strategies there is potential to "make the whole greater than the sum of its parts" (Walsh & Downe, 2005, p. 208). Through synthesis, qualitative research can become more potent, powerful, and accessible as evidence to inform occupational science and occupational therapy practice (Gewurtz, Stergiou-Kita, Shaw, Kirsh, & Rappolt, 2008; Pearson, 2004; Sandelowski & Barroso, 2002).

What is a meta-synthesis?

In response to the drive for evidence-based practice, specific processes for conducting systematic literature reviews have emerged and gained popularity (Taylor, 2007). These processes involve searching for the literature in a systematic and accountable way so that the search can be replicated if necessary. Typically, this systematic search process is guided by a review question which has a clearly identified population, intervention, comparison, and outcome. Using this method, the search terms and databases to be used are planned in advance and provided for the reader, along with the number of studies found during the search process (Grimmer-Somers, Kumar, Worley, & Young, 2009). In quantitative research, the findings from these studies are then extracted, re-analyzed, and reported in a narrative review or a meta-analysis.

A comparable process for managing and reporting findings from multiple qualitative research studies is to prepare a 'meta-synthesis'. A meta-synthesis approach involves systematically finding, reviewing, appraising, and bringing together findings of multiple qualitative research studies (Erwin, Brotherson, & Summers, 2011). The meta-synthesis product is a translation of the studies into each other. When you first encounter this idea as a novice to meta-synthesis the statement poses quite a challenge. What does it mean and how do we do that? The researcher has to take the themes, concepts, or metaphors from each study and transfer them across to the other studies. We describe the process of how we went about that translation later in the chapter. The outcome of a meta-synthesis is a combination of the findings from different studies, but at a higher conceptual level which could not be achieved with single studies alone and which is far more interpretive than the traditional descriptive narrative literature review. The utility of outcomes credited to the meta-synthesis process is growing in popularity and rigor (Gewurtz et al., 2008; Major & Savin-Baden, 2010).

History and development of meta-synthesis

The pioneers of the meta-synthesis approach in anthropology were Noblit and Hare (1998b) who called it a meta-ethnography. Their meta-ethnography involved seven phases and is used and cited extensively (Tatano Beck, 2009). The phases give guidance for comparing, synthesizing, and translating the "concepts, themes and phases of the findings" (p. 705) from the individual studies into third-order constructs, which are the resultant views and interpretations of the synthesis team about the topic: the desired endpoint (Malpass et al., 2009). Concurrent with the emergence of the meta-ethnography methodology was the emerging popularity of systematic reviews and meta-analysis in professional practice (Taylor, 2007). Contemporary methods for meta-synthesis in health science more closely mirror the systematic review process of identifying a review question, developing inclusion and exclusion criteria, systematically identifying studies, appraising those studies, and then synthesizing findings (Gewurtz et al., 2008).

Since the inception of the meta-synthesis approach there has been a yearning for clear guidelines and consensus regarding how to go about doing a meta-synthesis (Bondas & Hall, 2007). One of the difficulties with navigating the meta-synthesis literature is the lack of consistency of methods and variability of language used. However, it has been consistently concluded that meta-syntheses are interpretive rather than aggregative as is the case with meta-analysis (Finfgeld, 2003).

Our exploration uncovered that interpretive meta-synthesis involves lifting of the data to a more abstract or theoretical level, whereas a descriptive synthesis of the literature keeps the data contained in summaries. Descriptive approaches have different names in the literature including descriptive synthesis (Evans, 2002), textual narrative (Lucas, Baird, Arai, Law, & Roberts, 2007), and qualitative meta-summary (Sandelowski & Barroso, 2007). Of the more interpretive approaches, meta-ethnography (Tatano Beck, 2011), meta-synthesis (Finfgeld, 2003), qualitative research synthesis (Sandelowski, 2006), and qualitative evidence synthesis (Hannes & Macaitis, 2012) appeared to have similar steps. Variances in approach were dependent on the number of studies available about a topic, the quality of the studies, the detail provided in the studies about theoretical and methodological orientation, and how the findings were reported. Some authors claim that it is not sufficient to only extract and synthesize the study findings and propose that underlying theoretical and methodological orientations should also be compared and combined in a 'meta-study' (Finfgeld, 2003; Paterson, Thorne, Canam, & Jillings, 2001; Sandelowski & Barroso, 2007). However, we concluded that there are no clear rules about how it should be done; therefore, the researcher conducting the meta-synthesis needs to clearly explain and justify the methods selected.

Much of the literature about using a meta-synthesis approach is written for researchers exploring topics with a substantial quantity of literature for inclusion, leaving scholars in a smaller field unsure how to adjust the approach to suit their needs. In occupational science and occupational therapy, meta-synthesis approaches that allow for combining of findings with different methodological approaches (i.e. grounded theory, phenomenology), and smaller numbers of appropriate studies about a topic, is probably more feasible.

Epistemology

The epistemology of meta-synthesis needs to be congruent with the aim of generating a broader model or theory from the synthesis that is not possible from smaller studies or just one study. As we see and use meta-synthesis, it fits within an interpretive paradigm. Postmodern critiques of meta-synthesis are concerned about the model or theory that is generated being taken as 'one truth' or one 'true' account. Rather, situated in the interpretive paradigm, the aim is to deepen our understanding and generate a theory which as Walsh and Downe (2005) stated "is always transitory and open to revision, because phenomena are mutable and fluid" (p. 205). Further, Zimmer (2006) argued that the synthesized account across methodologies may place meta-synthesis as a particularly postmodern approach.

Having made the claim that meta-synthesis is situated within an interpretive paradigm, an astute reader would probably be able to detect some positivist undertones or overtones. The whiff of positivism probably arises because of the meta-synthesis being viewed as a qualitative version of the systematic review. The systematic review process of enumerating every step of the literature search process and processes of reducing bias in the review by researchers independently conducting searches or critically appraising articles and then making sure that they can reach consensus are examples of a more positivist approach to the study.

Acknowledging the nod to positivism, we will be describing an interpretive meta-synthesis approach that we believe to have utility in an occupational science and occupational therapy context. To illustrate our suggested approach for a meta-synthesis, we will draw on our experience and examples of meta-syntheses from the occupational therapy literature.

The review question

The first stage of an interpretive meta-synthesis is to decide on a clearly articulated review question about a topic aiming for a new theoretical understanding of the research findings. Establishment of the topic under investigation and the ensuing question is pivotal to development of the most appropriate review method. The topic for our study came from our interest in establishing what was already known about the transition from being a clinician to an academic (Murray et al., 2013). We knew that there was scant research from occupational therapy but were curious to learn what had been published in other related professions. The question guiding our review process was, "How do academics in nursing and allied health experience the transition to higher education from clinical roles?"

Examples of review questions from studies specific to occupational therapy include "What are mental health consumers' experiences and viewpoints regarding finding and keeping employment in integrated workplaces?" (Fossey & Harvey, 2010), "What is the experience of engaging in occupation following stroke for older people living in the community?" (Williams & Murray, 2013), and "What is the influence of the environment on participation for adults living with chronic disease?" (Hand, Wilkins, Letts, & Law, 2013).

Search terms and search strategy

Once the topic and review question are decided, the search for appropriate literature can begin. To make this search systematic and transparent to the reader, it is necessary to decide in advance the databases to be searched and the search terms to be used (Grimmer-Somers et al., 2009). Search terms can have truncations to capture all variations (e.g., clinic* will capture any term beginning with those 5 letters such as clinician(s) and clinical). Carolyn's search terms were academ* OR facult* AND transition, and the search was further refined by adding the terms qualitative AND clinic* OR practit* OR profession*. A preliminary search to see what literature is available and to get a sense of the journals that commonly publish the kind of studies being searched for and keywords that are used is useful at this point. If the search yields no results, then the topic will need to be broadened. Similarly if the search has too many results such as in the thousands, limits and refiners will need to be used.

The search process is not a straight linear process as it appears in the reporting of searches in the literature but involves a more recursive process until a manageable size selection of studies is found. What is manageable will depend on the scope of the review, the richness of the findings, and the purpose, but based on our experience somewhere between 5 and 15 studies for an honors student and 20–35 studies for a PhD student is acceptable. We found it helpful to enlist the support of an academic librarian who has sophisticated working knowledge of the best databases to search and can assist with keyword selection and limit setting.

A decision needs to be made about whether to include 'grey literature' such as reports on websites and unpublished doctoral theses. We decided not to include grey literature as it has not been peer reviewed and is difficult to search for in a systematic way. Another decision is whether to include narrative systematic reviews which have already been done about the chosen topic. This will depend on the scope of the project and the amount of literature available, but our experience has been that it is more straightforward to only include primary qualitative research studies.

The inclusion and exclusion criteria will help with planning the scope of the study and need to include details about the population of interest and the topic being explored. One of the key inclusion criterion will be that the study being searched for is qualitative. Each criterion for inclusion needs to be justified giving transparent reasons for the selections. For example, in Carolyn's meta-synthesis of the experience of transition from clinician to academic, the inclusion criteria included details of how long the new academic had been in the role. This criterion was supported by research found during the preliminary scoping of the literature and what was considered an appropriate amount of time for academics to be able to look back on but still remember their experience. The inclusion criteria also provided a detailed list of the disciplines for inclusion within the review in order to keep the meta-synthesis within scope and to find comparable experiences. If Carolyn had wanted to broaden her meta-synthesis, she could have included teachers or engineers, as there was some literature available from these disciplines.

Keeping the review tight and within scope ultimately made it easier to target a journal later for publication. However, during the process of developing inclusion and exclusion criteria, it is necessary to maintain a reflexive stance and be sure that all appropriate studies are being included even if their findings conflict or contrast with the main ideas on the topic. It is possible that translation of studies that are 'outliers' from the rest of the findings will make the process more challenging, but that is not a justifiable reason for exclusion of the study. Thus, a balance is required in keeping within topic and scope but also being rigorous in the process and managing the data that are available.

During the search and data extraction phases, it is necessary to keep track of how many studies are found in each database, how many duplicates are removed, and the screening process for refining the number of studies for inclusion in the meta-synthesis. This process is similar to that recommended by PRISMA group for quantitative systematic reviews and meta-analyses (Moher, Liberati, Tetzlaff, & Altman, 2009) and is helpful to the reader if presented in a flow chart such as Figure 12.1.

Critical appraisal of the included studies

Once the studies have been selected for inclusion in the review, it is necessary to appraise the quality of each one. If a study is deemed to be of poor quality, it may be excluded from the review at this point.

In our attempts to appraise the qualitative studies included in our meta-synthesis, we found that existing tools, such as the McMaster Critical Review Form (Letts et al., 2007) or the CASP qualitative research tool (CASP International Network, 2010), were applicable to qualitative research published in clinical and health journals which have a consistent approach for reporting research studies. However, due to the nature of our topic being the transition from clinician to academic, the studies we were appraising were published in educational journals which did not appear to contain the level of information about methodology and rigor that we were used to. As a result, there was a mismatch between the studies we were appraising and the detailed and prescriptive nature of the critical appraisal tools available to us. During attempts to critically appraise qualitative research, Gewurtz and colleagues (2008) warned researchers about unnecessarily excluding rich and useful studies from meta-syntheses due to inappropriate quality criteria being applied as will be discussed later in the chapter.

To appraise the literature in our study, we first reviewed the methods used in other meta-syntheses published in high-quality journals and found variability in stance about the need for quality appraisal and the subsequent approach used (Levack, Nicola, & Fadyl, 2010; Salter, Hellings, Foley, & Teasell, 2008; Whalley Hammell, 2007). Second, we read the general literature about how to read and interpret qualitative literature (Finfgeld-Connett, 2010; Sandelowski & Barroso, 2002; Santy & Kneale, 1999) and re-read some of the seminal pieces in the research methodology literature (Krefting, 1991; Patton, 2002). Following the process of weighing up the options, it seemed a commonly accepted method was to develop criteria that were a fit to the topic and the type of research being appraised (Cohen & Crabtree, 2008); hence, we decided to use a more topic-specific approach rather than attempting to apply rigid and prescriptive criteria. We modified an approach used by Salter et al. (2008) using the two headings of 'credibility' and 'relevance'.

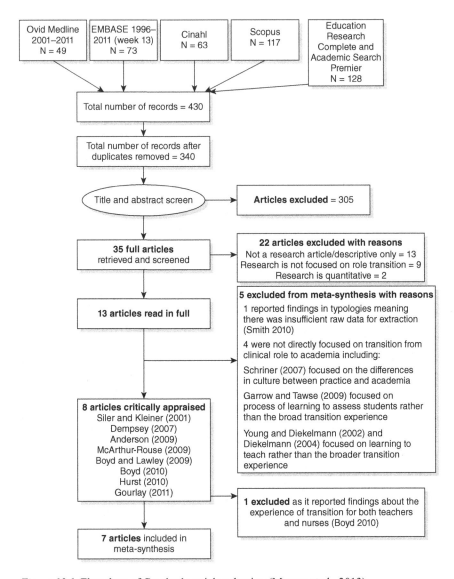

Figure 12.1 Flowchart of Carolyn's article selection (Murray et al., 2013)

We also added 'neutrality' due to the potential power issues around researchers interviewing academic colleagues in their own workplace. Credibility refers to the 'truth value' of a study, which is an assessment of how well it reflects the experience of the participants. The findings should have a resonance for the participants and for the reader. To appraise relevance, the question asked is "Has enough information been given to judge the influence of the researcher's biases and assumptions on the study?"(Krefting, 1991). In Textbox 12.1, we list the questions that we asked in relation to each rigor criterion.

Textbox 12.1   Appraising rigor

Credibility

1   Does the researcher explain the process of recruitment and data collection?
2   Does the researcher explain the process of data analysis?
3   Do the findings reported involve thick description?

Relevance

4   Are the characteristics of the participants described?
5   Does the author give suggestions for future research?
6   Are the findings related back to the research context?

Neutrality

7   Is there evidence of reflexivity being used by the researcher?
8   Does the researcher explain the relationship to the research participants?
9   Are limitations stated about the research?

Where there is sufficient research to do so, another approach is to have over-riding criteria in addition to existing critical appraisal tools. For example, Williams and Murray (2013) used the 10 questions of the CASP critical appraisal tool (CASP International Network, 2010) but also developed two additional criteria of 'having an auditable research process' meaning there was sufficient detail provided about how the research was conducted and that 'sufficient raw data were reported in the findings' so that data extraction was fruitful. These two criteria were essential indicators for making a decision about study inclusion in the meta-synthesis after critical appraisal. In a similar position of having many studies to draw into her meta-synthesis, Whalley Hammell (2007) incorporated the work of five different scholars in developing her eight criteria related to transferability, appropriate choice of methods, plausibility, and data quality. Other authors have used the critical appraisal approach described by Henderson and Rheault (2004) which draws on Guba's model of trustworthiness of data, as most of the qualitative appraisal tools do; however, we find some of the explanations and examples of criteria within their framework to be limited in the understanding of qualitative research. Where Henderson and Rheault's framework differs is in the assignment of studies to a hierarchy of evidence based on responses to the appraisal of trustworthiness. This assignment to levels of evidence is common within evidence-based practice drawing on effectiveness studies but not within qualitative work.

For rigor, Carolyn appraised all articles, and we divided the appraisal task between the two supervisors/co-authors. We compared the outcomes and had discussions until consensus was reached on the appraisal.

Data extraction and analysis methods

For our review about the transition experience from allied health clinician to academic, we made a few important decisions at the beginning. The first decision was to do a meta-synthesis rather than a meta-study given the small number of studies. This decision meant that we only extracted and synthesized the research findings of the studies and not the theories and methods (Evans, 2002; Major & Savin-Baden, 2010; Sandelowski & Barroso, 2007). The second decision was to exclude grey literature as we wanted to include research that had been critically appraised through peer review. Having said that, we found that the quality of the seven studies was not high, but we decided to include all the studies for extraction and secondary analysis as the findings were rich.

Data analysis for this study was conducted manually. Software programs such as NVivo can be used; however, our personal preferences is to actually 'handle' the data as this fit with our preferred ways of working. Information stored in a computer database that cannot be seen becomes invisible for people who are predominantly visual learners and thus can limit the cognitive flexibility required in good interpretive analysis. If the data set is very large, use of software is probably necessary and helpful for managing the data or could be suitable for researchers with different preferred learning styles.

Data analysis in our meta-synthesis involved three stages which involved taking the analysis through a first, second, and third order. The first order involves the basic concepts (or early codes), the second order involves the development of the constructs (categories), and the third order involves the lifting of the findings to a more abstract interpretation. The use of the notions of different levels of constructs is variable, but in our minds guides the development of new conceptual knowledge which is the desired endpoint of the meta-synthesis. Making the process transparent in the reporting adds rigor to the review (Classen, Winter, & Lopez, 2009). We will use the order framework to describe the analysis process for our review below.

The first-order analysis was to extract the findings from the seven studies and to print each of the findings onto different colored paper so any particular piece of data could always be traced back to its original source. Using this method, we organized the data into chunks which were coded and then spread pieces of coded data out over a large surface. Each individual code was then considered and compared to other codes. For example, codes that related to feeling like a novice or having to start again were placed together. Grouping similar codes together was an iterative process and continued until all codes were allocated to a cluster which became a category. Categories were allocated a tentative name (such as 'feeling new') that was descriptive of the content within the category. At this point, we kept the labels tentative so as to remain open to new interpretations of the data and to ensure they stayed as close to the content as possible. The development of categories marked the arrival at the second-order constructs of the meta-synthesis

While spreading out the data on the floor, dining table, desk, or whatever surface available assists the researcher, it is often not feasible or appropriate to leave the data out on display. The researcher can draw diagrams or take photographs to capture each stage of analysis but probably needs to have a system for storing data in between analysis sessions while maintaining where the analysis is 'up to'. We used a simple but effective system of ziplock plastic bags and yellow sticky notes which we jokingly refer to as "the Stanley tried and true plastic bag method". The sections of data are bagged up at the end of the analysis session and stored in a labeled plastic bag until the next session.

The process of constant comparison, examining each grouping, and comparing it to another grouping continued. During analysis we asked the questions, "What is this grouping about?" "How does it relate to the review question?" "How is it similar or different to all the other groupings?" Answering the questions or the process of debating the answers enabled us to further the analysis and draw relationships between the categories. Other questions to ask are "What does this say at a conceptual level?" and "How do I lift the data analysis to a higher order of abstraction without losing the 'life' in the themes?" This is the process of third-order interpretation and continues throughout the writing stage of the review and is more rigorous if discussed with peers. At this point it is also helpful to return to the original studies to check the interpretation remains consistent with, and is not too removed from, the original study findings.

The third-order analysis enabled us to conceptualize the four categories about the transition from clinician to academic as phases that new academics moved through before reaching their new identity. These phases were 'feeling new and vulnerable", 'doing things differently', 'expecting the unexpected', and 'evolving into the academic'. The phases took 1–3 years, and the change in identity became a central theme across the whole process. The higher level conceptualization of the data would have been challenging to justify on the basis of one small qualitative study alone and hence the translation of the seven studies into one provided stronger evidence about what the experience involved. The generic analysis process of meta-synthesis as described by Noblit and Hare (1998a) is presented schematically in Figure 12.2.

One of the contentious issues is the synthesis of studies that involve different qualitative designs. We questioned whether it was appropriate to combine findings of studies that originally had different epistemologies and ontologies. When

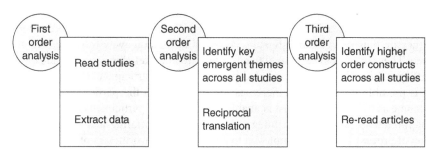

Figure 12.2 Schematic of the analysis process

we came to examine the different designs used by the researchers of the transition to being an academic studies this was not such an issue. Most of the studies made generic statements about the research design and indeed used a generic qualitative descriptive study design. On closer examination of the studies that stated a specific design when we conducted the quality appraisal we made a judgment that the study had not been conducted with strict adherence to the epistemological underpinnings of the design but rather was similar in design to the other studies and thus the findings could be comfortably synthesized.

However, the issue of synthesizing different designs continues to be debated in the methodological literature. Zimmer (2006) suggested that studies with either a grounded theory or ethnographic research design were readily synthesized as they share a common theoretical orientation, whereas phenomenological studies might be synthesized separately. Until that debate is resolved researchers will need to make their own decision based on the studies in front of them and explicate their reasoning in the review.

Rigor and ethics

The utility and transferability of a meta-synthesis will in part be dependent on the quality of the reporting in the original studies. The findings have to be presented in the original study in a manner which enables the researcher to extract data yet retain the richness of the data of the original study. Journal publication restrictions including word limits can restrict researchers from presenting the findings in a way that would be best for extracting for a meta-synthesis; however, journals would arguably say that the purpose of publication is not with meta-synthesis in mind. The researcher conducting the meta-synthesis needs to be mindful of the richness of the data they are including in the analysis and make sure that the findings are not too conceptually "thin" which will occur if the extracted data are sparse.

A further challenge to rigor is the increasing distance of the findings of the meta-synthesis from the original participants (Sandelowski, 2006; Walsh & Downe, 2005). The original data have been through a process of co-construction between the researcher and those researched and a level of interpretation. In the meta-synthesis, the data undergo a further co-construction between the interpreted data and the meta-synthesist, who further interprets the findings along with the findings of other studies. The findings of a meta-synthesis at a higher level order construct are thus moved through many layers of abstraction away from the original data. There is a risk at each level that the data are interpreted in ways that are quite different from the original intended meaning of the participants (Sandelowski). It is possible then that risk increases the further from the participants the data become as the meta-synthesist is unable to return to the participants to check their interpretations. Thus, rigor strategies such as peer debriefing and thick description of process need to be employed to ensure the trustworthiness of the findings.

Doing a meta-synthesis raises an interesting ethical dilemma. The participants of the original studies will have consented to their participation based on an informed consent process of reading an information sheet which outlined their rights, what their involvement in the study entails, and the risks that might arise from participation. They did not consent to their data being used for a meta-synthesis. There is little risk of participants' anonymity being compromised; however, the person conducting the meta-synthesis needs to be mindful of what the participants consented to. Every effort must be made to arrive at useful higher order constructs which advance knowledge and/or contribute to better occupational therapy practice in order to justify the lack of specific ethical clearance.

Critiquing studies

Given that there is little consensus about methods for conducting a meta-synthesis, critiquing studies is difficult. However, from our reading and experience we suggest the questions in Textbox 12.2 below as a guide to the critical reader.

Textbox 12.2   Critiquing studies using meta-synthesis

1   Has the *review question* been clearly stated?
2   Are the *inclusion criteria explicated and justified*?
3   Is the *search strategy* detailed, thorough, and comprehensive?
4   Are the *procedures for data extraction and analysis* clear?
5   Are strategies that were used to ensure rigor provided?
6   Have the authors *justified procedural decisions* such as combining studies with different designs?
7   Do the outcomes of the synthesis provide *new conceptual understandings*?
8   Is the synthesis useful?
9   Is the synthesis succint and elegant?

Application to occupational science

The findings from the meta-synthesis contribute to knowledge about occupational transitions and changes in occupational identity. The majority of studies of transitions in occupational science have focused on populations with a particular ill health condition such as stroke, or the transition of becoming a parent or retiring from paid employment (Nayar & Stanley, 2014). The findings from our meta-synthesis about the transition to academia add knowledge about a non-clinical population situated in the everyday.

While much of the research in occupational science is qualitative, the science may not be old enough or advanced enough to have a sufficient pool of research studies to draw on, or the studies may be too disparate, to conduct a meta-synthesis. However, in some areas it is likely that there are a number of studies that could be collated around a concept, for example, occupational adaptation. Meta-synthesis of studies around concepts in occupational science will advance the science and reveal gaps in knowledge which can be used to guide future research directions. Alternatively, researchers can conduct a meta-synthesis of studies in a related field and analyze the data through an occupational lens. Both of these approaches offer potential for occupational science.

Application to occupational therapy

The majority of studies we included in the meta-synthesis were from nursing, with one study from the physiotherapy profession. Thus, collating the studies for the meta-synthesis revealed a gap in knowledge about the transition for occupational therapy academics and provided a strong rationale for the need for Carolyn's honors research study. Despite the gap in occupational therapy, specific knowledge of the findings are still potentially useful for occupational therapists given that elements of the transition experience are likely to be common. The experience of new academics in finding themselves very unsettled and uncertain and having difficulty with finding and understanding the tacit knowledge in the foreign cultural environment of the university may be reassuring for others knowing that it is a common experience. It appears that up to 3 years are needed to adapt to the new culture and to make a shift in identity. The findings provide some guidance for strategies for prevention of frustration and disillusionment, and support of the academic, particularly with the adoption of the full academic role and the balancing of complex demands. Our experience with conducting a meta-synthesis provides support for the usefulness in revealing gaps in knowledge and in providing direction for researchers and for students who seek a research topic in an area where knowledge generation is needed.

Authors' reflection

In Carolyn's experience, doing the meta-synthesis made the development of method and analysis of the data of her subsequent study easier. Working through the critical appraisal process of studies that were similar to the one being planned enabled Carolyn to reflect about methods of rigor to employ to ensure that the flaws as identified in existing research were avoided. Being immersed in the topic gave greater clarity about where the gaps were in existing knowledge. When analyzing data from the subsequent study, it was necessary to avoid allowing the findings from the meta-synthesis to overlay the emergence of new findings and to make clear distinctions during analysis about what was new and what was unique to the occupational therapy participants and context. For Mandy, the attraction of meta-synthesis came from the view of it offering a qualitative alternative to a systematic review. The opportunity to build on knowledge generated in small studies and to build theory by combining smaller studies bringing the commonalities together is very appealing.

Meta-synthesis is best suited to those with some experience in qualitative research, particularly analysis. We believe it would be a much greater challenge for someone to move through the first-, second-, and third order constructs and lifting the data to a higher level of abstraction at the third-order level without having previous experience of qualitative analysis. In our view, and experience, it is an approach that is well suited to researchers working as a pair or in a small team.

Conclusion

For students or researchers, conducting a meta-synthesis is one approach to bringing together the published literature. Following methodological guidelines provides a structured, rigorous approach which is potentially publishable. There is no one way to conduct a meta-synthesis, and indeed there is a lot of confusion evident which may well stem from the use of the word synthesis, given that it is also commonly used to describe a related but different process of reporting what is already known about a particular field. However, the confusion of the range of approaches is not very different from the range of ways a researcher can approach, for example, grounded theory, or phenomenology or discourse analysis as explained in earlier chapters. Each researcher must read widely and make a decision about the approach they are going to take based on what feels like a good match with personal style and on exemplars that appeal in the published literature. In a sea of knowledge gaps, meta-synthesis offers an approach to connecting islands of knowledge to contribute to a great knowledge land mass.

References

Bondas, T., & Hall, E. O. C. (2007). Challenges in approaching metasynthesis research. *Qualitative Health Research, 17*(1), 113–121. doi:10.1177/1049732306295879.

CASP International Network. (2010). *Critical skills appraisal skills programme: Making sense of the evidence.* Retrieved from http://www.casp-uk.net/about-casp

Classen, S., Winter, S., & Lopez, E. D. S. (2009). Meta-synthesis of qualitative studies on older driver safety and mobility. *OTJR: Occupation, Participation and Health, 29*(1), 25–31.

Cohen, D. J., & Crabtree, B. F. (2008). Evaluative criteria for qualitative research in health care: Controversies and recommendations. *Annals of Family Medicine, 6*(4), 331–339.

Erwin, E. J., Brotherson, M. J., & Summers, J. A. (2011). Understanding qualitative meta-synthesis: Issues and opportunities in early childhood intervention research. *Journal of Early Intervention, 33*(3), 186–200. doi:10.1177/1053815111425493.

Evans, D. (2002). Systematic reviews of interpretive research: Interpretive data synthesis of processed data. *Australian Journal of Advanced Nursing, 20*(2), 22–26.

Finfgeld, D. L. (2003). Metasynthesis: The state of the art – so far. *Qualitative Health Research, 13*, 893–904.

Finfgeld-Connett, D. L. (2010). Generalizability and transferability of meta-synthesis research findings. *Journal of Advanced Nursing, 66*(2), 246–254. doi:10.1111/j.1365-2648.2009.05250.x.

Fossey, E. M., & Harvey, C. A. (2010). Finding and sustaining employment: A qualitative meta-synthesis of mental health consumer views. *Canadian Journal of Occupational Therapy, 77*(5), 303–314.

Frank, G., & Polkinghorne, D. (2010). Qualitative research in occupational therapy: From the first to second generataion. *OTJR: Occupation, Participation and Health, 30*(2), 51–57.

Gewurtz, R., Stergiou-Kita, M., Shaw, L., Kirsh, B., & Rappolt, S. (2008). Qualitative meta-synthesis: Reflections on the utility and challenges in occupational therapy. *Canadian Journal of Occupational Therapy, 75*(5), 301–308.

Grimmer-Somers, K., Kumar, S., Worley, A., & Young, A. (2009). *Practical tips in finding the evidence: An allied health primer.* Manila, Philippines: UST Publishing House.

Hand, C., Wilkins, S., Letts, L., & Law, M. (2013). Renegotiating environments to achieve participation: A metasynthesis of qualitative chronic disease research. *Canadian Journal of Occupational Therapy, 80*(4), 251–262. doi:10.1177/0008417413501290.

Hannes, K., & Macaitis, K. (2012). A move to more systematic and transparent approaches in qualitative evidence synthesis: Update on a review of published papers. *Qualitative Research, 12*, 402–442. doi:10.1177/1468794111432992.

Henderson, R., & Rheault, W. (2004). Appraising and incorporating qualitative research in evidence-based practice. *Journal of Physical Therapy Education, 18*(3), 35–40.

Krefting, L. (1991). Rigor in qualitative research. *American Journal of Occupational Therapy, 45*(3), 214–222.

Letts, L., Wilkins, S., Law, M., Stewart, D., Bosch, J., & Westmorland, M. (2007). *Critical review form: Qualitative studies* (version 2). Retrieved from http://www.srs-mcmaster.ca/Portals/20/pdf/ebp/qualreview_version2.0.pdf

Levack, W. M., Nicola, M. K., & Fadyl, J. K. (2010). Experience of recovery and outcome following traumatic brain injury: A metasynthesis of qualitative research. *Disability and Rehabilitation, 32*(12), 986–999. doi:10.3109/09638281003775394.

Lucas, P. J., Baird, J., Arai, L., Law, C., & Roberts, H. M. (2007). Worked examples of alternative methods for the synthesis of qualitative and quantitative research in systematic reviews. *BMC Medical Research Methodology, 7*, 4–7. doi:10.1186/1471-228-7-4.

Major, C., & Savin-Baden, M. (2010). *An introduction to qualitative research synthesis: Managing the information explosion is social science research.* New York, NY: Routledge.

Malpass, A., Shaw, A., Sharp, D., Walter, F., Feder, G., Ridd, M., & Kessler, D. (2009). 'Medication career' or 'Moral career'? The two sides of managing antidepressants: A meta-ethnography of patients experience of antidepressants. *Social Science and Medicine, 68*, 154–168. doi:10.1016/j.socscimed.2008.09.068.

Moher, D., Liberati, A., Tetzlaff, J., & Altman, D. G. (2009). Preferred reporting items for systmatic reviews and meta-analyses: The PRISMA statement. *PLoS Med, 6*(6), e1000097.

Murray, C., Stanley, M., & Wright, S. (2013). The transition from clinician to academic in nursing and allied health: A qualitative meta-synthesis. *Nurse Education Today, 34*, 389–395. doi:10.1016/jnedt.2013.06.010.

Nayar, S., & Stanley, M. (2014). Occupational adaptation as a social process in everyday life. *Journal of Occupational Science.* doi:10.1080/14427591.2014.882251.

Noblit, G. W., & Hare, R. D. (1998a). *Meta-ethnography: Synthesising qualitative studies.* Newbury Park, CA: Sage.

Noblit, G. W., & Hare, R. D. (1998b). *Meta-ethnography: Synthesising qualitative studies.* Newbury Park, CA: Sage.

Paterson, B. L., Dubouloz, C. J., Chevrier, J., Ashe, B., King, J., & Moldoveanu, M. (2009). Conducting qualitative metasynthesis research: Insights from a metasynthesis project. *International Journal of Qualitative Methods, 8*(3), 22–33.

Paterson, B. L., Thorne, S. E., Canam, C., & Jillings, C. (2001). *Meta-study of qualitative health research: A practical guide to meta-analysis and meta-synthesis.* Thousand Oaks, CA: Sage.

Patton, M. Q. (2002). *Qualitative research and evaluation methods* (3rd ed.). Thousand Oaks, CA: Sage.

Pearson, A. (2004). Balancing the evidence: Incorporating the synthesis of qualitative data into systematic reviews. *JBI Reports, 2*, 45–64.

Salter, K., Hellings, C., Foley, N., & Teasell, R. (2008). The experience of living with stroke: A qualitative meta-synthesis. *Journal of Rehabilitation Medicine, 40*, 595–602. doi:10.2340/16501977-0238.

Sandelowski, M. (2000). Whatever happened to qualitative description? *Research in Nursing and Health, 23*, 333–340.

Sandelowski, M. (2006). 'Meta-jeopardy': The crisis of representation in qualitative meta-synthesis. *Nursing Outlook, 54*(1), 10–16.

Sandelowski, M., & Barroso, J. (2002). Reading qualitative studies. *International Journal of Qualitative Methods, 1*(1), 74–108.

Sandelowski, M., & Barroso, J. (2007). *Handbook for synthesizing qualitative research.* New York, NY: Springer.

Santy, J., & Kneale, J. (1999). Critiquing qualitative research. *Journal of Orthopaedic Nursing, 3,* 24–32.

Tatano Beck, C. (2009). Metasynthesis: A goldmine for evidence-based practice. *AORN Journal, 90*(5), 701–710. doi:10.1016/j.aorn.2009.06.025.

Tatano Beck, C. (2011). A metaethnography of traumatic childbirth and its aftermath: Amplifying causal looping. *Qualitative Health Research, 21*(3), 301–311. doi:10.1177/1049732310390698.

Taylor, M. C. (2007). *Evidence-based practice for occupational therapists* (2nd ed.). Oxford: Blackwell.

Tomlin, G., & Borgetto, B. (2011). Research pyramid: A new evidence-based practice model for occupational therapy. *American Journal of Occupational Therapy, 65*(2), 189–196.

Walsh, D., & Downe, S. (2005). Meta-synthesis method for qualitative research: A literature review. *Journal of Advanced Nursing, 50*(2), 204–211.

Whalley Hammell, K. (2007). Experience of rehabilitation following spinal cord injury: A meta-synthesis of qualitative findings. *Spinal Cord, 45,* 260–274. doi:0.1038/sj.sc.3102034.

Williams, S., & Murray, C. (2013). The experience of engaging in occupation following stroke: A qualitative metasynthesis. *British Journal of Occupational Therapy, 76*(8), 370–378. doi:10.4276/030802213X13757040168351.

Zimmer, L. (2006). Qualitative meta-synthesis: A question of dialoguing with texts. *Journal of Advanced Nursing, 53*(3), 311–318.

Further reading

Atkins, S., Lewin, S., Smith, H., Engel, M., Fretheim, A., & Volmink, J. (2008). Conducting a meta-ethnography of qualitative literature: Lessons learnt. *BMC Medical Research Methodology, 8*(21), 1–10.

Doyle, L. H. (2003). Synthesis through meta-ethnography: paradoxes, enhancements, and possibilities. *Qualitative Research, 3*(3), 321–344.

Erwin, E. J., Brotherson, M. J., & Summers, J. A. (2011). Understanding qualitative meta-synthesis: Issues and opportunities in early childhood intervention research. *Journal of Early Intervention, 33*(3), 186–200.

Mays, N., & Pope, C. (2000). Qualitative research in health care: Assessing quality in qualitative research. *British Medical Journal, 320*(1), 50–52.

Noblit, G. W., & Hare, R. D. (1988). *Meta-ethnography: Synthesizing qualitative studies.* London, UK: Sage.

Sandelowski, M., & Barroso, J. (2003). Classifying the findings in qualitative studies. *Qualitative Health Research, 13*(7), 905–923.

Thorne, S., Jensen, L., Kearney, M. H., Noblit, G., & Sandelowski, M. (2004). Qualitative metasynthesis: Reflections on methodological orientation and ideological agenda. *Qualitative Health Research, 14,* 1342–1365.

13 Appreciative inquiry

Enabling occupation through the envisioning mind

Jenni Mace, Clare Hocking, and Marilyn Waring

Textbox 13.1 Jenni's story

Not so long ago, Jenni was working with a mother living in temporary accommodation. As a refugee in a new country, the mother was unsure how she was going to provide for her children once she moved into a more permanent accommodation. She wanted to work but felt she had little education and few employable skills. Jenni asked her, if she could dream of a life with no barriers in her way, what job she would choose to do. Her reply was child care. Jenni smiled and looked at the mother's two healthy children playing nearby, and together they started writing down what she did well as a mother. It was not long before they had a long list of skills she could bring to a job in child care. The mother left that day imagining new possibilities for her future.

Working with clients to help them recognize their hidden talents and capabilities, beyond deficits, is not a new concept for occupational therapists. For individuals and groups who have faced enduring challenges in everyday life, recognition of strengths can lead to renewed aspirations. A strengths-based approach, informed by positive psychology, fits well with appreciative inquiry. This widely published research methodology is a type of action research that studies the positive aspects of a group, when it is working at its very best, in order to imagine and create positive change for the future (Cooperrider & Whitney, 2005). Despite the fit between practice and research, evidence of occupational scientists or occupational therapists using appreciative inquiry as a research methodology is sparse.

Fundamental to appreciative inquiry is the belief that in every group there is something positive that can be focused on, and this focus becomes a reality (Cooperrider & Whitney, 2005; Hammond, 1998). In Jenni's work in the housing and homelessness sector, she had seen the skills people use for daily survival on the streets or in hostels, such as resourcefulness, negotiating and caring for others, overshadowed by a focus on solving problems (Homeless Link, 2009). Encouraging these hidden strengths can lead to individuals seeking new positive directions for their future. It is this fact that has led Jenni to embark on her doctoral studies, which will involve partnering with a service provider to explore what they do well to help homeless families resettle and re-engage in the everyday routines associated with a place called home. Walking alongside Jenni are her doctoral supervisors and co-authors Clare Hocking, with her knowledge of occupational justice, and Marilyn Waring, with expertise in policy, human rights and supervising students using appreciative inquiry.

In this chapter, we propose that appreciative inquiry fits well with contemporary thinking in occupational science and occupational therapy, and is a useful tool for discovering strengths and imagining and generating new productive ways of doing and being. In the poetic spirit of appreciative inquiry, we will draw on metaphors and stories to illustrate the potential of appreciative inquiry as a method for occupation-focused research.

Background: the appreciative eye

Appreciative inquiry was developed by David Cooperrider in the early 1980s. Cooperrider's wife Nancy, an artist, drew his attention to an appreciative lens by pointing out that in art something beautiful can be found in every painting (Hammond, 1998). If attention is not drawn to the beautiful, it can be missed. In the same manner, Cooperrider proposed that if people focus on the problems in a situation or organization, they are magnified at the expense of what is already working well (Bellinger & Elliott, 2011). In the appreciative inquiry process, the future is developed through a focus on the core strengths of what or who is to be studied. This positive core is the means and ends of appreciative inquiry research (Cooperrider, Whitney, & Strovos, 2008).

Appreciative inquiry research has predominately been used in organizational development as a method of change management focusing on what works and why (Reed, 2007). There is also a growing body of research in education, health and social care using appreciative inquiry (Carter, 2006). The essential beliefs that guide an appreciative inquiry research project are its five core principles (Watkins & Mohr, 2001), which are explained below.

The constructionist principle

This principle upholds that relationships and human discourse are at the center of knowledge (Cooperrider & Whitney, 2005). Conversations give meaning to everyday life. The words people share are vital: they bring to life the world as we know it (Whitney &Trosten-Bloom, 2010). For instance, the word 'home' can simply be a description of the four walls people live within. However, when the meaning of home is discussed and shared in a group, it becomes a source of identity, security, belonging, memories or a center of people's occupations (Moore, 2007). The concept of home is constructed and brought to life by the shared words and ideas used to describe it.

The principle of simultaneity

Inquiry and change happen simultaneously (Cooperrider & Whitney, 2005). Inquiry is defined as exploring future potential through the act of asking questions and is viewed as an intervention that has the power to move change in a positive direction (Cooperrider et al., 2008). Positive change becomes a part of the inquiry. Therefore, the key to appreciative inquiry is asking questions that stimulate new visions for the future (Whitney & Trosten-Bloom, 2010).

The anticipatory principle

This principle is integral to encouraging participants to believe that the future will have better outcomes, so that they will act hopefully and positively in the present (Reed, 2007). Cooperrider et al. (2008) described anticipation as similar to sitting in front of a movie screen on which images of a wonderful future are being projected. Excitement is created, along with an anticipation that it is worth engaging in activities that will bring those images into reality.

The poetic principle

This principle views organizations, communities or individuals as open books with many plotlines, characters and settings. Researchers can choose to study any topic within the individual or shared narrative. Appreciative inquiry looks for the positive stories and helps the characters with the authoring and co-authoring of their book (Bushe, 2011; Cooperrider & Whitney, 2005; Reed, 2007). Metaphors are often used to organize common story lines and to create images of alternative futures.

The positive principle

In appreciative inquiry studies, it is argued that a focus on what people do well is more engaging and motivating, and that change is more likely to be sustained than in a study that focuses on what is going wrong (Watkins & Mohr, 2001). For example, in running a resettlement group with older homeless men, Jenni came to realize that the greatest sustainable change came from finding out the past trades and skills group members had before living on the street, and encouraging them to share those with other group members. Change seldom came from staff teaching group members' skills, which implies group members lacked them.

In these principles, it is important to note the underlying influence of discourse and narrative theories. Storytelling is an essential component of the appreciative inquiry process, especially at the start, where the positive and life-giving themes of collective narratives are discovered.

Epistemology

Appreciative inquiry straddles the qualitative and quantitative paradigms. It has an interest in the quality of experience and how people feel and think about what they do. However, because appreciative inquiry is a process where change might occur, it is often evaluated using quantitative measures. Ideas are tried out and consequences examined; the major difference being that ideas are tried out by the participants and planned as the project progresses. In this respect, appreciative inquiry deals with naturally occurring phenomena rather than controlled structured environments.

A number of authors describe appreciative inquiry as a methodology, a philosophy and a world view (Neumann, 2009; Watkins & Mohr, 2001). It has its own sets of principles, assumptions and processes designed to engage human systems in change. Change is seen as a continual process, occurring in every action and inquiry undertaken in order to understand or 'know' something about the world. While appreciative inquiry is a philosophy of knowledge, it also aligns with a variety of guiding theories (Watkins & Mohr).

Social constructionism

Appreciative inquiry is strongly grounded in social constructionism, particularly Kenneth and Mary Gergen's concept of generative theory (Bushe, 2011; Zandee & Cooperrider, 2008). Generative theory is a critical stance that challenges taken-for-granted knowledge (Watkins & Mohr, 2001), particularly assumptions about the way things happen (Reed, 2007). This in turn allows for the generation of new ideas and directions for social action.

Appreciative inquiry further emphasizes shared constructions of meaning and knowledge. Social interactions and language use within relationships are seen as a source of truth, helping to create the world as different individuals know it. This idea is used in appreciative inquiry through interviews and group work where ideas are explored and challenged with others (Gergen & Gergen, 2008; Reed, 2007; Watkins & Mohr, 2001). As individuals develop an understanding of their world, not only do their constructed thoughts and feelings change, so too do their actions and behaviors (Reed 2007; Watkins & Mohr, 2001).

Pragmatism

The main concern of pragmatism is to measure knowledge by what works (Cutchin & Dickie, 2012). Arguably this positive focus makes it one of the more obvious choices to guide appreciative inquiry research. Pragmatism is also constructionist in that it challenges taken-for-granted ideas and is therefore a theory that sits well with appreciative inquiry's epistemological roots (Crotty, 1998).

One pragmatist that resonates strongly with the principles of appreciative inquiry, and is increasingly discussed in the occupational science literature, is John Dewey. According to Dewey's transactional theory, people do not act independently of their environment in order to function; instead, there is a dynamic interaction and transaction of the individual with their environment. Dewey stressed that meaning making happens with all participants involved and is connected implicitly to the social environment. Dewey rejected dualisms, noting that rather than individuals being separate from society, despite their unique characteristics, they are thoroughly shaped by future opportunities arising from their context, including their language, culture, community and family (Cutchin, Aldrich, Bailliard, & Coppola, 2008; Frank, 2011). Thus, Dewey's ideas mirror appreciative inquiry's beliefs around group work, planning for the future and its social constructionist leanings.

Critical theory

Some appreciative inquiry authors also suggest a critical appreciative inquiry approach (Cockell & McArthur-Blair, 2012). Taking a critical theory approach might seem contradictory alongside the ever positive appreciative inquiry (Grant & Humphries, 2006). However, being critical does not mean being negative. For example, in inquiries such as those exploring homelessness, it would be difficult to imagine research not also aimed at improving issues of social justice and equality (Cockell & McArthur-Blair, 2012).

Grant and Humphries (2006) argued that critical theorists, including Derrida, Foucault and Lyotard, not only challenged social realities but aimed to facilitate change and promote human potential. These philosophers urged researchers to reflect on the taken-for-granted ideas and power of organizations, and how power differentials can be perpetuated through the use of language. This reflexive process can give voice to those who are not always heard (Grant & Humphries, 2006; Reed, 2007).

In New Zealand cities, as in many countries, lack of housing is a major issue; yet, the stories of those living and working with these issues are seldom told. The philosophical ideas touched on above are important tools to enable a group of people, such as the organizations that work with homeless families, to reflect and seek meaning in their actions for an enriched future.

Defining the topic and the positive question

Cooperrider et al. (2008) contended that appreciative inquiry researchers should start with investigating what gives vibrancy to the organization or situation and, using affirmative bold hunches, develop a topic or research question that focuses on these energizing factors. This process is referred to as the affirmative topic choice or choosing the unconditional positive question.

Developing an affirmative topic should encourage participants to move in a positive future direction. Defining a positive topic is important to the research process as it is what mobilizes a positive inquiry. It is essential that all participants are engaged and see the research as important, in order to elicit stories of success around the topic and visions of an ideal future (Watkins & Mohr, 2001).

The main purpose of Jenni's study is to explore what works well when providing services that will enable families in temporary accommodation resettle into a permanent home. Policy makers looking to end homelessness can only speculate at present on what works as this is a topic that has not been researched formally in New Zealand. Therefore, the main unconditional positive question guiding the research is, 'What makes the transition to sustaining a permanent home possible for families in temporary housing?'

Recruitment and sampling

Jenni's study is being carried out with an organization providing services to families in temporary accommodation. Six to ten families will join the study as experts to assist in the process and share the wisdom they gained from being successfully rehoused by that organization. Sampling in appreciative inquiry is purposive, in that participants are selected based on their knowledge of a population or organization and what works well. The organization being worked with is known for its success in helping families resettle in permanent homes.

Sampling is also driven by the concept of wholeness, in that it is important to include all key players in the organization or social group so that decisions made during the appreciative inquiry change process are supported by all the people those changes will effect in the long term (Reed, 2007). In a small organization, it may be possible to include everyone; for larger organizations, the amount of data and time required are not always practical. Fitzgerald, Murrell and Newman (2001) named three additional forms of qualitative sampling that help maintain the wholeness of the data and manage the amount of data.

Maximum variation sampling ensures that participants are selected to maximize diversity in the search for the positive. If an important contributor to the organization or diversity in families is missing, then an opportunity to discover new knowledge, understanding and innovative collaborative action may be compromised (Ludema & Fry, 2008). Extreme or deviant case sampling can also ensure that diversity is maintained and new knowledge is not lost. Jenni has worked with the management team to ensure staff members who want to be involved and can provide diverse and rich information are included.

Opportunistic or emergent sampling is used to take advantage of knowledge gained in the process of collecting data (Ludema & Fry, 2009). As the knowledge of the setting grows, Jenni will take advantage of unfolding events that could lead to other stakeholders who might extend knowledge by being invited to participate, especially in the latter phases of the appreciative inquiry process. However, people who may be important theoretically may not be seen as key players by the organization, and it is essential that the appreciative inquiry researcher listens to participants so that sampling can be collaborative (Reed, 2007).

Key staff members will help identify families who have been rehoused for 6 months or more, as they will hold some of the knowledge about what makes the transition to sustaining a permanent home possible. What constitutes a family has also been considered carefully, with an emphasis on residing in the same household and a social, rather than biological, connection. This allows for maximum variation and different types of parents to be included, for instance, natural, adopted, grandparents, step, same sex, foster or adults in a parental role (Hodgson & Birks, 2002).

Data collection

The principles of appreciative inquiry fit well with the characteristics of an emergent design, where the detail of the process and methods change and evolve to make the most of newly emerging issues, or unearth previously hidden knowledge (Hesse-Biber & Levy, 2008). That means the initial proposal cannot be too prescriptive as the participants will have input at each stage in the study, which demands flexibility (Creswell, 2009).

Action research

Many of the identifying features of appreciative inquiry are also features of action research (see Chapter 8). Action research has challenged the traditional idea of the researcher standing back from what is being studied, on the basis that the researcher can never be fully independent of the research environment (Reed, 2007). Additionally, because participants are encouraged to be co-researchers, they are able to evaluate their own environments and suggest new ways of enhancing their lives. The power of the researcher is leveled and communities are empowered through a process of investigating, reflecting, feedback, diagnosis and acting on their discoveries (Reed, 2007). However, action research, as its very name suggests, has action as its key focus, particularly where action is required to fix an issue or problem (Boyd & Bright, 2007; Reed, 2007). Consequently, critiques of action research suggest there is a loss of wonder about what does work, and wondering can lead to theory. Thus, it is proposed that appreciative inquiry, with its ability to challenge the taken for granted, is capable of theorizing alternative ways of being (Zandee & Cooperrider, 2008).

The appreciative inquiry process

Appreciative inquiry has a clearly defined cyclical process. While several variations are available to choose from, the most widely used framework is called the 4-D process (Watkins & Mohr, 2001), consisting of the discovery, dream, design and destiny stages (see Figure 13.1). More recently, some authors have added a fifth D, starting the process with 'define' (or 'topic choice'), which has been discussed above.

Discovery

This phase is about the best of what is (Elliot, 1999). It draws on as many stakeholders from the organization, team or group as possible to identify and analyze what gives life to their work or situation through appreciative interviewing and storytelling. This story collecting is sometimes called appreciative inquiry conversations (Reed, 2007). Individual stories of success are shared, either with the researcher or peers. Other activities can be used to elicit information about what works, including written accounts, observations, use of statistics or documents, photography, drawing or dramatization (Reed). Analysis is collaborative, aimed

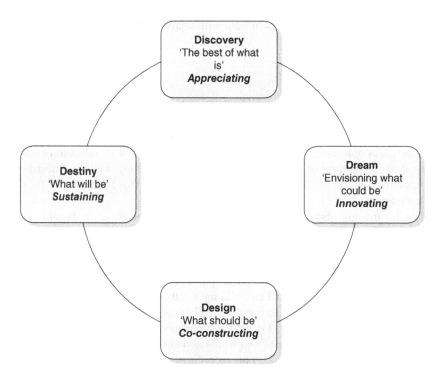

Figure 13.1 Appreciative inquiry 4-D cycle (adapted from Ludema & Fry, 2008)

at identifying common themes. A number of methods can be used to facilitate analysis, such as nominal group techniques for large workshops. This is where members share ideas such as 'what works well'. Ideas are recorded and duplicate ideas eliminated. Members then vote on the ideas that best represent their organization, so that collective themes become evident (Reed, 2007).

Jenni's research will use the cyclical process twice, beginning by using the wisdom of families who have successfully resettled, to identify what made the transition to a permanent home possible, before incorporating this information into the second process with service providers. The process used with families is focused on here in more detail to provide an example of how the four phases work. Families consent to being involved in the research after being fully informed that the information they provide will be fed-back to the organizations that helped house them. For the discovery phase, questions put to both groups have been influenced by the literature review and explore what shapes New Zealand meanings of home; for example, the objects that give occupants and the home identity, the occupations engaged in at home and the people who share that space. The concept of a treasure box holding the family's most precious things will be introduced. Family members will be asked to write or draw objects, people and activities that gave their family hope for the future. Next, by discussing the contents of their treasure box, they will develop a core list of things they agree gave them hope and kept them together as a family. Recordings of discussions within the families will help with analysis of common ideas across the families in the study.

Dream

The dream phase is about the best of what can be in the future (Carter, 2006). Participants imagine their organization or group functioning at its best (Preskill & Coghlan, 2003). The themes and stories from the discovery phase are used to develop ideas of a preferred future. This can be done through visualization exercises, drawing pictures of the future (Watkins & Mohr, 2001) or telling futuristic stories (Boyd & Bright, 2007). Themes are drawn out of these activities to form collective visions.

Having thought about what worked for families in the past, the families in Jenni's study will then be asked to dream about the future. First, on their own, and then together, family members will draw and discuss their ideal home and the occupations they do there. This information will be important to share with service providers when they do the dream phase, so that they can consider what is most important to families when building a stable home. After sharing their ideas, the family will be asked to combine the best of their ideas and design their collective dream family home. Lewis, Passmore and Cantore (2011) suggested making a montage of the pictures and words and adding magazine cuttings. The montages and collective drawings, plus recordings of joint discussions, will help with analysis of the data across families.

Design

The design phase is about planning and determining what will be. The ideas created from the dream phase are developed by members of the organization or group into strong actionable visions for the future (Ludema & Fry, 2008; Preskill & Coghlan, 2003). These future visions are referred to as provocative propositions and are assertive, confident and ambitious statements with no ifs or buts added (Reed, 2007). These statements are developed collaboratively, which past studies have found effective in decreasing hierarchy or inequality (Watkins & Mohr, 2001). Broad objectives on how to achieve these aspirational ideas and what resources are needed to carry them out are also developed and combined to make an overall strategy.

Members of the family will be asked: "If you were the boss of the organization that helped your family, what would you do differently in the future so other families can find a home that would help them to do what they want to do and be who they want to be?" The members of the family will then share their ideas with each other, drawing their ideas into the most important themes. These messages will be provocative propositions or visionary goals that can then be fed-back to service providers, so that they can be taken onboard for future planning.

Destiny

At this stage, it is suggested that others who might have a role in carrying out the objectives set in the design phase are invited to join in the process. If numbers allow, participants are put into groups that have the provocative proposition that they want to help achieve. Each group works on specific actions and assigns tasks that will help to achieve the objectives. It is important at this point to make sure someone in the organization, other than the researcher, will follow up to ensure plans are implemented and evaluated (Lewis et al., 2011).

The closing activity with families will be to discuss who, other than the organization that helped rehouse them, needs to hear their provocative statement and what actions should be taken to deliver these ideas. For instance, what do they think needs to be done to achieve these ideas? To complete the 4-D process and allow families to receive some personal benefit from their involvement, the montages of their ideal home will be presented to them. It will be suggested that they work together to develop three achievable goals to pursue that will help them continue to improve their home and family life.

It is at this point families will also be given the option to take their collective ideas and themes to the organization and assist Jenni using similar creative activities to help the housing providers, dream, design a plan and create provocative propositions about how they envision they will work with families in the future. This will enable families who have experienced successful resettlement to see their concerns and ideas being harnessed and used in a positive way.

Data analysis: mining for the hidden gems

The data collection activities above allow for shared analysis through which stories of success are told in various ways and participants work together to extract and refine key themes. Group analysis has been designed to allow all members within a group to be heard, further enabling decision making at each stage to be auditable and transparent.

In some studies, especially where more than one group is involved, further thematic analysis alongside interpretive reflexivity is carried out. Researchers look for hidden themes that do not emerge from group discussion, critically review ideas and search for new meaning (Reed, 2007). It is important to note here that additional themes discovered by the researcher need to be checked by participants in order to maintain a collaborative and transparent approach.

A model of analysis that fits both the ethos of appreciative inquiry and the focus of the research has been chosen. Clandinin and Connelly (2000) proposed a narrative analysis called the three-dimensional space approach. What makes their analysis appropriate is that it is based on Dewey's philosophy of experience and much of appreciative inquiry is based on storytelling and narrative (Reed, 2007). The three dimensions in this approach are interaction, continuity and situation (Ollerenshaw & Creswell, 2002). Group data and transcriptions of recorded discussions are thematically mapped and analyzed around these three major concepts.

Interaction

This involves the researcher mining the data for both the personal and the social experiences of the storytellers. The personal information may include hopes, dreams, emotions and moral dispositions. Social information includes the interaction between people, existential conditions in the environment, and the views, assumptions and purposes of others. Social constructionist theories will apply here.

Continuity

The researcher looks for temporality within a text, analyzing the past, present and future. Temporality works well with appreciative inquiry as it gives the opportunity to highlight information from the best of what is and was (discovery), plus data related to the future (dream, design and destiny).

Situation

Using Dewey's ideas of situation, any settings where a problem or enjoyment is experienced, resulting in an event (Frank, 2011), will be extracted from the data. Of particular interest is how problematic situations influence occupations and transaction with the environment in positive ways (Cutchin & Dickie, 2012).

To demonstrate the analytic process, we draw on a quote from a strengths-based study that sought to identify the ways well-being was experienced in the lives and occupations of people in Australia who were homeless (refer to Table 13.1) (Thomas, Gray, & McGinty, 2012). That study included homeless families, and this particular quote illustrates how well-being is maintained through the occupations of a mother. We have analyzed it from the perspective of Jenni's research question: What makes the transition to sustaining a permanent home possible for families in temporary housing?

> Just basically keep on with my normal life as it is at the moment, trying to keep my children in a routine as much as possible, so that they have got a cushioning, so that they can at least fall back on their routine, that they know I am still there and things are still the same, that's not going to change. And that gives them the sense of security even though they are not living where they were before. (Alex)

Clandinin and Connelly (2000) discussed the process of sorting field texts into the three categories, interaction, continuity and situation, as part of an archival process that includes narrative coding of dates, contexts, characters and topics discussed. Field data are read and re-read in order to narratively code characters, storylines and plots that interconnect. As summarized in Table 13.1, analysis involves restorying the data, which needs to be checked by participants to stay true to the essence of what they are trying to say (Ollerenshaw & Creswell, 2002). Clandinin and Connelly further stated that in order for the research text to be socially significant and meaningful, theory, literature and the research question itself must be revisited when moving from fieldwork to final analysis.

Table 13.1 Illustrative example of the analytic process

Interaction		Continuity			Situation
Personal	Social	Past	Present	Future	
Keeping on with normal life and routines are important to Alex	Alex provides a cushioning by carrying out familiar routines together as a family	They lived in a different place from now	Maintaining routines now allows the children to have a feeling that at least there are two constant things in their lives that will not change; Alex and their routines	Alex and the family routines will stay with them into the future	For Alex, what works for her family in a new living situation is maintaining familiar family routines Or – Alex and her children have been through a time of upheaval and loss. As far as she can, she wants to protect them from any negative impacts
Alex hopes to keep things the same and that there is a sense of security, something to fall back on	The kids know their mum is still there for them, despite other things changing				

Rigor and ethics: looking into the shadows

Reflexivity

Reed (2007) noted that while analysis is vital to making sense of and organizing the data so that it is accessible to others, the process should not stop there. Ideas need to be critically reviewed and alternative or new ways of thinking generated through thoughtful reflection. By its very nature, appreciative inquiry does this, especially in organizations where those things that should be appreciated are neglected. Fitzgerald, Oliver and Hoxsey (2010) discussed appreciative inquiry's ability to highlight the overlooked through Jung's concept of the shadow: those things that are suppressed, denied or considered inappropriate. Putting a spotlight on what is going well means that people who are not normally acknowledged will be. Therefore, appreciative inquiry can be used to draw out the hidden positives of people or organizations.

Fitzgerald et al. (2010) argued that because of its uncompromising focus on the positive, the negative can be swept into the shadows. Therefore, the researcher needs to be aware of what might be lurking there. The shunned, censored or denied ideas need to be reflexively listened for and acknowledged, before being able to proceed successfully with an appreciative focus. By completely ignoring the negative, what people have learnt from those experiences might be missed. The appreciative inquiry literature encourages transparency and honesty with participants and has examples of how to overcome barriers on the day (Fitzgerald et al., 2010). What 'shadows' are not observed and dealt with in the presence of participants can be captured through the use of reflective models and diaries; discussion with supervisors or peers is another method. To avoid personal bias, researchers also need to keep a critical eye on the values and preconceived ideas they bring to the research and how that influences the way they interpret what they see, hear and read (Etherington, 2004).

Audit trails

Reed (2007) contended that appreciative inquiry studies are often complex, multifaceted and multilayered; hence, researchers need to maintain a clear and structured audit trail. At each stage of the process, it needs to be obvious how themes were developed and the decisions that led to them. Transcripts and reflective diaries are useful tools for recording decisions made.

Trustworthiness

While reflexivity and a transparent audit trail will contribute to the trustworthiness of the findings, other qualities built into the design will also help. Triangulation can assist in trustworthiness through multiple methods of data collection such as storytelling, group discussion and drawings. Triangulation can also be gained through multiple sources of data, for example, staff, clients and family. Member checking data with participants throughout is essential.

Critiquing appreciative inquiry

Appreciative inquiry is not without its critics, and there are limitations that threaten to derail the processes and integrity of this methodology. Fitzgerald et al.

(2001) described these as mythical dragons and suggested methods for slaying them. These dragons are introduced below, along with newer beasts.

The scaredy-cat dragon

Possibly the most prominent dragon, this beast is mistakenly known for its ability to hide behind a rosy take on life, ignoring the harder issues. As described above, the appreciative inquiry literature does not encourage researchers to ignore the challenges that lurk in the shadows. Past studies acknowledge that ignoring the negative can decrease involvement in the process. Exploring negative contexts with an appreciative eye can lead to finding creative and overlooked alternatives. Positive questions can be asked, such as, what have issues taught us that make us better at what we do? On the few days when things went well, what made the difference? Appreciative inquiry authors argue that behind every negative story lies a positive (Bushe, 2011; Reed, 2007).

The warm fuzzy dragon

While often leaving a room full of happier people, this dragon is not always taken seriously. It might be easy to perceive that such an approach to research lacks quality and rigor. Despite the differences in data collection methods and approach, appreciative inquiry has many processes in place in its pursuit of rich qualitative data and is often supported by quantitative data. Warm and fuzzy as it may appear on the outside, the inner workings of appreciative inquiry are very rigorous (Fitzgerald et al., 2001).

The big fat dragon

With its focus on the whole, especially in sampling, appreciative inquiry projects can be very big and long. Participants may move on or ideas can become stale in the course of data collection. It is important to give this careful consideration in the design and analysis of an appreciative inquiry project (Bellinger & Elliot, 2011).

The blinkered dragon

Appreciative inquiry projects may be blinkered to power dynamics (Reed, 2007). If appreciative inquiry is pushed by managers, there may be subtle pressure in the direction they want it to go. Having managers present may also influence what is said. This is of course part of a socially constructed world, but again design needs to be considered when reflecting on how the overlooked point of view can be heard. Textbox 13.2 poses questions to ask when reviewing studies claiming to use appreciative inquiry methodology.

**Textbox 13.2   Critiquing appreciative inquiry studies –
questions to ask**

1   Is there a clear affirmative, topic choice and *unconditional positive
question*?
2   Is the study underpinned by social constructionism and the *appreciative inquiry principles*?
3   Are the methods underpinned by the *4-D process*? Is it clear that the
research has actively sought out the best of what is and what could be?
4   Are *stories of success* shared?
5   Has the sampling been driven by the *concept of wholeness*, including at
least the key players that will be impacted by any resulting change?
6   Have *research decisions*, including analysis, been *made collaboratively* with participants?
7   Does the researcher *demonstrate reflexive practice*?

Application to occupational science

A core assumption of occupational science is that there is a relationship between health and engagement in occupation or meaningful activity for individuals, families, communities and populations (Wright-St Clair, 2012). Needing to know how and why action occurs is central to understanding occupation and its relationship to well-being. It is also central to the pragmatic concern for what works (Cutchin & Dickie, 2012). There is logic to choosing appreciative inquiry in asking what occupations contribute to a fulfilling and healthy life.

In a similar vein, positive psychologists study positive emotions and how they contribute to well-being. Emerging alongside and supporting appreciative inquiry, the science of positive psychology has developed out of the observation that psychology has largely focused on the negative emotions and their impact on health (Cockell & McArthur-Blair, 2012). Walley Hammell and Iwama (2012) made a similar observation in the occupational science literature, stating that while occupational scientists assume a positive connection between well-being and occupation, research to support this is minimal. Appreciative inquiry would seem a logical choice to advance this research in order to answer questions about what works, such as what occupations enable people to flourish and why?

Application to occupational therapy

Occupational therapists have many of the skills required to be effective appreciative inquiry practitioners, as reflected in recent occupational therapy literature. As a profession, they are experts at eliciting stories from clients about the challenges and issues of daily life and capable of turning the focus on to strengths and resources in order to enable occupation (Townsend & Polatajko, 2007). The profession's client-centered ethos enables occupational therapists to partner with clients in analyzing and reflecting on the strengths in their narratives; in the same way that appreciative inquiry is uncompromisingly collaborative (Townsend & Polatajko, 2007). Thomas et al. (2012) advocated strongly for strengths-based approaches, such as appreciative inquiry, in order to reveal hidden life experiences, occupations and community capacity. Townsend and Polatajko (2007) recognized appreciative inquiry as a requirement for the enablement of occupations. They pointed out that occupational therapists, like appreciative inquiry researchers, appreciate the often taken for granted or overlooked activities of daily life, especially when asking questions such as 'what do you do or want to do that is meaningful to you?'

Personal reflection: the waking dream

Jenni's choice to use appreciative inquiry for her doctoral studies reflects her practice as an occupational therapist, which draws upon a strengths-based approach (see Textbox 13.1). Practicing from within this paradigm, Jenni strives to enable hope for all those with whom she works. Hope is a quality characterized by a vision for new possibilities despite current challenges. In helping participants dream of a different future, appreciative inquiry can help foster hope. Hope is magical, as it feeds people's motivation and self-efficacy and gives them the courage to try new things (Cockell & McArthur-Blair, 2012).

Being without a home threatens a hopeful future (Partis, 2003). However, in Jenni's work in the field of homelessness and in the literature, we continue to discover evidence of hopelessness turned around, and not always by providing a house. As stated in the introduction, making individuals aware that they have strengths and capabilities is vital, and this is often achieved through engaging people in occupations that are meaningful to them (Fisher & Hotchkiss, 2008; Petrenchik, 2006).

Summary

This chapter has taken the reader along a path of an appreciative eye, philosophical guides, hidden treasure, dark shadows, dragons and hope for a happy ending. However, unlike the fairy-tale metaphor, we suggest appreciative inquiry is a methodology that has a solid foundation in theory and rigor, and takes itself very seriously. As demonstrated above, it shares many of the current values and beliefs of both occupational science and occupational therapy. Appreciative inquiry has the potential to provide evidence of the positive contributions both disciplines are making in our communities and to promote ongoing healthy occupational change in the populations we work alongside.

References

Bellinger, A., & Elliot, T. (2011). What are you looking at? The potential of appreciative inquiry as a research approach in social work. *British Journal of Social Work, 41,* 708–725. doi:10.1093/bjsw/ber065.

Boyd, N., & Bright, D. (2007). Appreciative inquiry as a mode of action research for community psychology. *Journal of Community Psychology, 35*(8), 1019–1036.

Bushe, G. (2011). Appreciative inquiry: Theory and critique. In D. Boje, B. Burnes, & J. Hassard (Eds.), *The Routledge companion to organizational change* (pp. 87–103). Oxford, UK: Routledge.

Carter, L. (2006). Home and location: The problem of place as an ethnic identifier. *International Journal of the Humanities, 4*(3), 33–44.

Clandinin, D., & Connelly, F. (2000). *Narrative inquiry: Experience in story in qualitative research.* San Francisco, CA: Jossey-Bass.

Cockell, J., & McArthur-Blair, J. (2012). *Appreciative inquiry in higher education: A transformative force.* San Francisco, CA: John Wiley & Sons.

Cooperrider, D., & Witney, D. (2005). *Appreciative inquiry: A positive revolution in change.* San Francisco, CA: Berrett-Koehler Publishers.

Cooperrider, D., Whitney, D., & Stravos, J. (2008). *Appreciative inquiry handbook: For leaders of change* (2nd ed.). Brunswick, OH: Crown Custom Publishing.

Creswell, J. (2009). *Research design: Qualitative, quantitative and mixed methods approaches.* Los Angeles, CA: Sage.

Crotty, M. (1998). *The foundations of social research: Meaning and perspective in the research process.* London, UK: Sage.

Cutchin, M. P., & Dickie, V. (2012). Transactionalism: Occupational science and the pragmatic attitude. In G. E. Whiteford & C. Hocking (Eds.), *Occupational science: Society, inclusion, participation* (pp. 23–38).Oxford, UK: Wiley-Blackwell.

Cutchin, M. P., Aldrich, R. M., Bailliard, A., & Coppola, S. (2008). Action theories for occupational science: The contributions of Dewey and Bourdieu. *Journal of Occupational Science, 15*(3), 97–99. doi:10.1080/14427591.2008.9686625.

Elliot, C. (1999). *Locating the energy for change: An introduction to appreciative inquiry.* Winnipeg, Canada: The International Institute for Sustainable Development.

Etherington, K. (2004). *Becoming a reflexive researcher: Using ourselves in research.* London, UK: Jessica Kingsley Publishers.

Fisher, G. S., & Hotchkiss, A. (2008). A model of occupational empowerment for marginalized populations in community environments. *Occupational Therapy in Health Care, 22*(1), 55–71. doi:10.1300/J003v22n01_05.

Fitzgerald, S., Murrell, K., & Newman, H. (2001). Appreciative inquiry: The new frontier. In J. Waclawski & A. Church (Eds.), *Organization development: Data driven methods for change* (pp. 203–221). San Francisco, CA: Jossey-Bass Publishers.

Fitzgerald, S., Oliver, C., & Hoxsey, J. (2010). Appreciative inquiry as a shadow process. *Journal of Management Inquiry, 19*(3), 220–233. doi:10.1177/1056492609349349.

Frank, G. (2011). The transactional relationship between occupation and place: Indigenous cultures in the American Southwest. *Journal of Occupational Science, 18*(1), 3–20. doi :10.1080/14427591.2011.562874.

Gergen, K., & Gergen, M. (2008). Social construction and research as action. In P. Reason & H. Bradbury (Eds.), *The Sage handbook of action research: Participative inquiry and practice* (2nd ed., pp. 159–172). London, UK: Sage.

Grant, S., & Humphries, M. (2006). Critical evaluation of appreciative inquiry. *Action Research, 4*(4), 401–418.

Hammond, S. (1998). *The thin book of appreciative inquiry.* Bend, OR: Thin Book Publications.

Hesse-Biber, S., & Leavy, P. (2008). *Handbook of emergent methods.* New York: The Guilford Press.

Hodgson, R., & Birks, S. (2002). *Statistics New Zealand's definition of family, its implications for the accuracy of data effectiveness of policy targeting.* Palmerston North, New Zealand: Centre for Public Policy Evaluation, Massey University.

Homeless Link. (2009). *Policy briefing: engagement, education, training and employment.* Retrieved November 24, 2010, from http://homeless.org.uk/education-training-employment#.Ut3OJbH2–70

Lewis, S., Passmore, J., & Cantore, S. (2011). *Appreciative inquiry for change management: Using AI to facilitate organizational development.* London, UK: Kogan Page.

Ludema, J., & Fry, R. (2008). The practice of appreciative inquiry. In P. Reason & H. Bradbury (Eds.), *The Sage handbook of action research: Participative inquiry and practice* (2nd ed., pp. 280–296). London, UK: Sage.

Moore, J. (2007). Polarity or integration? Toward a fuller understanding of home and homelessness. *Journal of Architecture and Planning Research, 24*(2), 143–159.

Neumann, C. (2009). Appreciative inquiry in New Zealand: Practitioner perspectives. Unpublished thesis, University of Canterbury, New Zealand.

Ollerenshaw, J., & Creswell, J. (2002). Narrative research: Restorying data analysis approaches. *Qualitative Inquiry, 8*(3), 329–347.

Partis, M. (2003). Hope in homeless people: A phenomenological study. *Primary Health Care Research and Development, 4*, 9–19. doi:10.1191/1463423603pc118.

Petrenchik, T. (2006). Homelessness: Perspectives, misconceptions, and considerations for occupational therapy. *Occupational Therapy in Health Care, 20*(3), 9–30.

Preskill, H., & Coghlan, A. (2003). Using appreciative inquiry in evaluation. *New Directions for Evaluation, 100*(Winter), 5–99.

Reed, J. (2007). *Appreciative inquiry: Research for change.* Thousand Oaks, CA: Sage.

Thomas, Y., Gray, M., & McGinty, S. (2012). An exploration of subjective wellbeing among people experiencing homelessness: A strengths-based approach. *Social Work in Health Care, 51*(9), 780–797. doi:10.1080/00981389.2012.686475.

Townsend, E., & Polatajko, H. (2007). *Enabling occupation II: Advancing an occupational therapy vision for health, well-being & justice through occupation.* Ottawa, Canada: Canadian Association of Occupational Therapists ACE.

Walley Hammell, K., & Iwama, M. (2012). Well-being and occupational rights: An imperative for critical occupational therapy. *Scandinavian Journal of Occupational Therapy, 19*, 385–394. doi:10.3109/11038128.2011.611821.

Watkins, J., & Mohr, B. (2001). *Appreciative inquiry: Change at the speed of imagination.* San Francisco, CA: Jossey-Bass/Pfeiffer.

Whitney, D., & Trosten-Bloom, A. (2010). *The power of appreciative inquiry: A practical guide to positive change.* San Francisco, CA: Berrett-Koehler Publishers.

Wright-St Clair, V. (2012). The case for multiple research methodologies. In G. E. Whiteford & C. Hocking (Eds.), *Critical perspectives on occupational science: Society, inclusion, participation* (pp. 137–152). Oxford, UK: Blackwell Publishing.

Zandee, D., & Cooperrider, D. (2008). Appreciable worlds, inspired inquiry. In P. Reason & H. Bradbury (Eds.), *The Sage handbook of action research: Participative inquiry and practice* (2nd ed., pp. 190–198). London, UK: Sage.

Additional resources

AI practitioner: An international journal of appreciative inquiry. Retrieved July 15, 2014, from http://www.aipractitioner.com/

Appreciative inquiry commons: A worldwide portal for sharing AI academic resources and tools. Retrieved July 15, 2014, from http://appreciativeinquiry.case.edu/

Kelm, J. (2011). *What is appreciative inquiry?* Retrieved July 15, 2014, from http://www.youtube.com/watch?v=ZwGNZ63hj5k

Myrada Project. (2011). *Appreciative inquiry: A beginning.* Retrieved July 15, 2014, from http://www.youtube.com/watch?v=pVBMMJ0RMao

14 Interrogating power and reason

Critical theory and philosophy

Ben Sellar

I am sitting in a workshop that addresses issues of sex, gender, identity, and discrimination in therapeutic work. I have enjoyed these workshops for their assertion that practice is a political issue. Having been trained in anatomy, physiology, psychology, kinesiology, splinting, home modifications, and wheelchair prescription, I welcome this critical approach to the work. I suspect others have welcomed it too. Each week my classmates and I have enthusiastically aligned ourselves to the workshop material with remarkable unanimity. Yes, I am against violence to women! Yes, homophobia is a horrendous injustice! Yes, racism is something that I understand and actively work against in the community! But strangely, with every performance of agreement I become increasingly suspicious that I do not agree at all. Rather, I feel that I am guarding against exposure as an ally of male entitlement, heteronormativity, and white privilege. So today, when everyone agrees that sexual difference is the socially constructed effect of power relations I clumsily tender my dissent:

> But some things aren't constructed. When I watch cricket I would rather watch men play, because they hit the ball harder, bowl the ball faster, and take more diving catches. Men's sport is better to watch because men actually are stronger and faster.

This comment is met with outrage.

I feel myself redden. No doubt I have exposed myself, but something else is going on. The critical and political value of the ideas in the workshop is clear and important. Yet they seem to come at the cost of well-established scientific facts about hormones and musculoskeletal structure that differentiate men from women. Are these facts social constructions? If so, does this undermine the value of my scientific training as an occupational scientist and therapist? If not, then what is my capacity for critical political engagement?

This experience introduced me to the difference between traditional and critical theory (although there are some common themes that most critical theorists agree on; see, for example, Table 14.1). Traditional theory had taught me the truth about sexual dimorphism in humans, but critical theory was showing me how this truth subordinated women to patriarchal ideas of strength and rationality. Traditional theory had taught me to be a dispassionate observer of the world,

Table 14.1 Traditional versus critical theory

	Traditional theory	Critical theory
Aims	Accurate representation of natural facts	Human liberation from oppressive ideology
Theory	Objective analytic propositions produced in isolation from sociohistorical conditions	Purposeful intervention into sociohistorical conditions
Truth	Product of scientific inquiry	Product of power relations
Researcher	Distanced and unbiased observer	Invested and reflexive actor
Validity	Repeatable method and falsifiable results	Greater self-understanding and self-direction for participants
Critique	Is this knowledge rigorous and thus a true representation of the facts?	How has this knowledge come to gain truth status and what is the effect?
Ontology	Objects exist outside of human knowledge	Objects exist outside of human knowledge
Epistemology	Good knowledge is that which conforms to objects	Good knowledge is that which understands that objects always conform to pre-existing human knowledge

but critical theory was showing me the importance of passionately intervening in the world to make it a better place. Traditional theory had taught me to look very closely at the object of analysis, but critical theory was teaching me to look very closely at myself, and the assumptions, values, and beliefs that shaped the way I came to see the object in the first place.

Previously, I had loved knowing the anatomical and physiological details of the human body so as to intervene effectively as a therapist. But now new questions began to matter. How have physical strength and speed become the criteria for "good" sport? How has the morphological complexity of humans been turned into a simple sexual binary and what are its effects? How have I come to be so invested in these patriarchal conditions and what can I do about it?

This story speaks partially of the problems that delivered me to critical theory and philosophy. In this chapter, I examine the role of critical theory as a research approach in occupational science and occupational therapy. Throughout, I will draw upon my doctoral work that examined how the dualism of science and politics operated in occupational justice to stave off the overwhelming complexity and subjective discomfort that such an idea should engender in a white, educated, minority male.

Background

> The philosophers have only interpreted the world in various ways; the point is, to change it.
>
> (Marx, 1888/1969, p. 15)

Marx's quote succinctly expresses the ambitions of critical theory. Marx had a problem with philosophers who took the existing state of affairs as natural, given, and only in need of interpretation. Despite its fame, this quote expresses a line of thought articulated by Immanuel Kant almost 100 years earlier. It is therefore useful to briefly discuss the critical philosophy of Kant, starting with an analogy.

Imagine a discussion between yourself and a mantis shrimp about the accuracy of a photograph. While swimming on a reef with friends you stop to take a photograph of the scene in front of you. You think the photograph accurately represents the scene because it includes every form, expression, color, and object that you can see yourself. But the mantis shrimp interjects and points out that it does not match what she sees. The mantis shrimp has at least 10 photoreceptors compared to your 3 (Cronin & Marshall, 1989; Cronin, Caldwell, & Marshall, 2001) and can see polarized light (Chiou et al., 2008). Compared to the 1 million gradations of color visible to you, the mantis shrimp sees 1,000,000,000,000,000,000,000,000 gradations, as well as colors that you cannot, and so she regards your picture as a gross simplification of the reefs complexity. So is the picture accurate or not?

The shrimp helps you to see that accuracy is relative. The photograph is not a neutral reproduction of the scene in front of you. It has been mediated by photographic structures including a lens, shutter, exposure time, and film to construct an image. Similarly, the scene has been mediated through your optical structure involving the eye, retina, visual cortex, and association areas to produce an image. The photograph and the image appear to correspond, because both the photographic and optical structures that mediate the scene filter the same light. The accuracy of the picture cannot be measured in isolation. The picture is accurate *for you*, and inaccurate *for the shrimp*. Both the photograph and your image of the reef are caricatures that foreground some characteristics and background others. All you can see of the reef is all that your optical structures allow you to see. You did not sense the inaccuracy of the photograph because your senses could not sense it. This seeming truism is important for Kant.

Despite not having his own mantis shrimp, Kant worried about the same problem. Many of Kant's contemporaries were empiricist philosophers who deduced knowledge of the world from their senses alone. Kant wondered, 'if we can only know things through our fallible senses, how do we know we have an accurate picture of the world?' Furthermore, 'if we only have access to our sense of the object, how can we be sure that there is an object there at all?' Kant argued that the empiricist position was limited not only by optical structures but knowledge structures in the human mind that similarly mediated their view of the world. He took space as a key example. The empiricists sought to carefully sense external objects to determine their objective characteristics. But Kant pointed out that we need only rely on our senses if space is like a big three-dimensional room in which the object and the observer occupy different Cartesian coordinates. That is, senses are assumed to mediate between the object over there and its representation in my mind. While such a notion of space seems commonsense, the empiricists could not prove it because any attempt at proof must presuppose it. So while empiricists considered sense to mediate between the world and the mind, empiricism itself was mediated by a presupposed concept of space that could not be empirically proven (see Textbox 14.1, point 1). The empiricists had encountered a paradox that they could not resolve.

Kant's response was to revolutionize the idea that human knowledge conforms to objects and to experiment instead with the hypothesis that objects conform to knowledge (See Textbox 14.1, point 3). Just as the accuracy of the image was relative to my optical structures, perhaps knowledge of objects was relative to my knowledge structures.

Textbox 14.1   Basic assumptions of critical theory

1   All thought is fundamentally mediated by power relations that are socially and historically constituted
2   Facts can never be isolated from the domain of values or removed from some form of ideological inscription
3   The relationship between concept and object and between signifier and signified is never stable or fixed and is often mediated by the social relations of capitalist production and consumption
4   Language is central to the formation of subjectivity (conscious and unconscious awareness)
5   Certain groups in society and particular societies are privileged over others and, although the reasons for this privileging may vary widely, the oppression that characterizes contemporary societies is most force-fully reproduced when subordinates accept their social status as natural, necessary, or inevitable
6   Oppression has many faces, and focusing on only one at the expense of others (e.g., class oppression versus racism) often overlooks the interconnections among them
7   Mainstream research practices are generally, although most often unwittingly, implicated in the reproduction of systems of class, race, and gender oppression

(Kincheloe, McLaren, & Steinberg, 2011)

Kant saw that by clarifying the knowledge structures mediating thought, we could make them available to transformation and enable progress beyond the limits of contemporary commonsense, just as I might use gene therapy to increase my visible spectrum (Mancuso et al., 2009). If transforming my optical structures seems extreme, imagine what might be possible if I transform my idea of space itself.

Kant's revolution had implications for social and political progress. He argued that reasonable social progress, that is progress lead by reason, could be achieved only if pre-existing knowledge structures were critiqued and their presuppositions exposed. Hegel inherited this legacy and pursued philosophy as "the movement of reason, the act of fully self-conscious thought that in its act reveals the contradictions latent in ordinary or natural understanding" (Stepelevich, 2010, p. 239). Post-Kantian philosophy began to position itself as an actor in the history and progress of reasonable society.

Marx explicitly stipulated that philosophers make an emancipatory intervention. He compelled philosophers to work with oppressed people to better understand their conditions and the powerful ideologies that shape them. Such clarity, he argued, would better position oppressed people to transform their conditions and effect their own emancipation. As such he defined critical theory as "the self-clarification of the struggles and wishes of the age" (Marx, 1975, p. 209).

"Self-clarification" was crucial for Marx because he saw that history was always written by those in power. "The ideas of the ruling class are in every epoch the ruling ideas" (Marx & Engels, 1970, p. 64). History was always an interpretation of human events made by those who won the battles, controlled the means of production, and sought to maintain power. The power to produce the dominant interpretation of world history was significant for two reasons. First, the ruling class had no motivation to transform the interpretation, and so transformative ideas would not come from them. Second, ideas were politically significant as a means of shaping social and political futures (see Textbox 14.1, point 3). Further, as state power was increasingly integrated into civil society, it became harder and harder to know where and how it was operating to shape people's worldview.

Foucault pursued deeply embedded forms of state power through studies of medicine (Foucault, 1963/1994), madness (Foucault, 1976/1978), criminality (Foucault, 1975/1977), and sexuality (Foucault, 1976/1978; 1984/1992; 1984/1990) to see how binaries such as sane/insane, lawful/criminal, and normal/deviant had become commonsense. By analyzing the relationship between informal knowledge (connaissance), as expressed through everyday activities (i.e., what is polite or impolite, reasonable/unreasonable, worthwhile, not worthwhile), and formal knowledge (savoir), expressed in scientific texts, philosophical theories, and religious justifications, he showed how such binaries came to appear as obvious and true. Foucault's (1997) contribution to critical theory is expressed to some extent in his essay *What is critique?* where he declares that

> . . . critique is the movement by which the subject gives himself [sic] the right to question truth on its effects of power and question power on its discourses of truth. Well, then!: critique will be the art of voluntary insubordination . . . the politics of truth. (p. 47)

For Foucault, then, critical theorists are insubordinates who voluntarily and explicitly disobey commonsense to examine how it has achieved truth status.

In my PhD study, I used Foucault extensively to question how occupational justice had been so unanimously endorsed as an intrinsically good direction for occupational science and occupational therapy. Implicating as it does such complex issues as rights, emancipation, oppression, colonialism, subjugation, capitalism, power, language, freedom, which are in themselves extremely complex and contested, how was it that no one was debating this new political project? My departure point then was to give myself the right to question the concept, to voluntarily stand as an insubordinate in order to examine the conditions that fostered consent to the idea, and how I was, myself, implicated.

This brief background shows that critical theory is interested in how knowledge is produced, what mediates or shapes that knowledge, how that knowledge affects people (especially those oppressed or subjugated by it), and what opportunities there are for transforming those conditions into the future. Such an emphasis on knowledge makes epistemology a key issue in critical theory.

Epistemology

Epistemology is extremely important to critical theorists who regard it as constituting first philosophy. Before inquiring about an object of knowledge, we must first examine our ways of knowing. For critical theorists, pre-existing knowledge structures function as tools for constructing knowledge and so, just as any construction worker does, critical theorists want to first inspect the fitness or suitability of these tools (Bryant, 2011). It is useful to explore what constructivism means, how it differs from social constructivism, and the constructive power of discourse and language.

Bruno Latour studied the practices undertaken to produce scientific facts in laboratories (Latour & Woolgar, 1986) where the artificiality of experimental science and the objectivity of scientific facts function alongside one another (Latour, 2005) without contradiction. Latour showed that constructing a fact does not make it unreal and so undermined debates between constructivists and realists in which "Either a fact is real or it's fabricated" (Latour, 2005, p. 91). Just like a building, facts are both real and fabricated. Constructing a building requires intensive work by a collective of humans and nonhumans whose respective properties and strengths are combined to produce something capable of withstanding relevant tests. Buildings are not judged for being real or constructed but by whether they are well or poorly constructed. Can it stand up to high-speed winds or earthquakes, use by people with disabilities or children, and ecological regulations?

Though at risk of oversimplification, this example subverts the dualism between real and constructed knowledge and does so at the very site where some of the most powerful truths are constructed (Latour & Woolgar, 1986). Hence, to construct knowledge is to make it stand, and this is not simple. Truth is not a direct effect of power, but power can be used to enroll the labor necessary to produce a construction that appears to stand as natural, true, and ironically, unconstructed. For critical theorists then, facts can never be separated from the values and ideas of those with the power to construct them (see Textbox 14.1, point 2). Such a view directs critique toward how well or poorly the knowledge is constructed. What has been assumed or presupposed? Who has been included or excluded in this construction? In what interests has it been constructed? What unanticipated effects is this construction having (Brown, 2004)? What tests reveal the limitations of the construction (Butler, 2004)? And, where are the opportunities for reconstructing it differently?

The second misunderstanding of constructivism concerns its habitual pairing with the word 'social' in such form as 'social constructivism', 'social constructions', or 'social constructs'. Such terms make it unclear how society or the social is itself constructed (Latour, 1988). Critics of reductionism in natural and biological sciences protest the reduction of complex phenomena to ever smaller elements; as said they are primary, causal, and more real. But appealing to 'social construction' performs the same reduction, only this time posits society as more primary, real, and causal than smaller elements (Harman, 2011). Latour (2005, p. 137) argued that appealing to "social forces" compensates for a poor description of those forces themselves or how society itself is constructed. Social constructivism compromises the validity of critical research by failing to adequately detail oppressive conditions and thus limiting its emancipatory potential.

Having discussed some basic tenets of constructivism, I now turn to the key tools for construction identified by various critical theorists. Marx argued that ideology obscured how the oppressed perceived reality because it was constructed and perpetuated by the daily habits and behaviors made necessary by capitalist industry, and so always served the needs of those in power. But as Zizek (1994) noted, ideology is a coherent doctrine or composite set of beliefs and concepts that convince us of their truth but may serve unacknowledged social or political interests. So ideology is not necessarily imposed but has the power to convince people such that they subscribe to it themselves.

Foucault (1969/2007) argued that people consent to power through the everyday linguistic, verbal, symbolic, and bodily acts that make up everyday life. These acts compose what he called discourse and serve as the conduit for power and knowledge. Take language as one powerful discursive element. The words and grammatical structures available to us force us to think in terms of a sovereign subject "I" because other forms are rendered insensible. While it is common to say "It is raining" without specifying what "it" is, similar language when describing a human action seems unintelligible. Thus, grammar and language posit an active doer behind the deed in a way that can obscure distributed or collective agency involving collectives of humans and nonhumans alike (Bennett, 2010). So language has the power to bring into being that which it appears to only represent (Austin, 1975) (see Textbox 14.1, point 4). In this case, language produces a sovereign, intentional individual agent that independently initiates or causes action.

Though language is a common site of analysis for critical theorists, different traditions will place greater emphasis on specific elements and mechanisms than others. What is common to all critical research is an explicit description of the epistemology adopted and appreciation that epistemology matters (Butler, 1993), that is, ways of knowing condition what matters. Where traditional theory derives its epistemology from an unstated ontology of prestructured objects in a container, critical research must give an account of how it understands knowledge to be constructed and how it participates in that construction itself. This is crucial if it is to limit the extent to which the research itself unintentionally perpetuates oppressive realities (see Textbox 14.1, point 7).

Choosing a question

For the critical researcher, the choice and wording of a question is always political as it determines who will be involved, whose interests are being taken up, and who will be left out. An unreflective approach to question design risks perpetuating the very norms and visibilities that reproduce systems of class, race, and gender oppression. Researchers need to justify their question in terms of its research validity and its political validity or its capacity to have an emancipatory effect. As conditions of oppression are multifaceted, then the question will need to be able to navigate the complex entanglements of various forms and histories of oppression (see Textbox 14.1, point 6).

Critical research questions typically involve two key aspects: something taken for granted and a group of affected people. First, the question will need to interrogate an idea, concept, practice, or behavior that is taken for granted as true, proper, good, and so forth. The researcher can then analyze the conditions of possibility for appearing as commonsense or obviously good. Second, the question examines how whatever it is that is being taken for granted affects particular groups. For example,

1   How do contemporary media constructions of retirees and retirement shape the possibilities and constraints for older people's being and doing? (Laliberte Rudman, 2005, p. 150)
2   How does the dualism of science and politics in occupational justice shape the legitimate political capacities of vulnerable people? (Sellar, 2012)
3   Does the notion of "women" deployed in feminist politics exclude from political representation those who do not fit with its heteronormative presuppositions? (Butler, 2006, p.7)

Each of these questions takes something that appears natural and given (retirement, science and politics, womanhood/feminism) and then interrogates its effects on a particular group (retirees, vulnerable groups, unrepresented people). Each question is explicitly political, concerned with knowledge production, and its role in designating legitimate subject positions.

Recruitment and sampling

Critical research seeks to produce detailed descriptions of the conditions affecting people. It thus privileges intensive samples, in which few cases are analyzed for multiple properties, over extensive samples, where few properties are analyzed across vast numbers of cases (Morrow & Brown, 1994). As such, sampling is thus typically purposive or theoretical and focused on critical cases that can "yield the most information and have the greatest impact on the development of knowledge" (Patton, 2002, p. 236). This means that sampling procedures should be chosen based on their consistency with the interpretive and analytic paradigms of the research.

Critical research very often involves the analysis of texts. In such cases, recruitment can be relatively straightforward but sampling must be carefully considered. Investigating occupational justice discourse, I limited the sample to published texts that had passed an editorial or peer-review process. From an initial literature review, I identified the texts of Wilcock and Townsend as critical cases. Through their rich exposition of the concept of justice, these texts provided fruitful connections to other disciplines and times, thus constituting an intense and productive point for entry into the discursive network.

Following Foucault's (1969/2007) archaeological method, subsequent texts were sampled iteratively by identifying connections between analyzed texts and others that operated in concert with them. Connections were made by examining which texts were used in the production of another, as well as what presuppositions remained unarticulated but necessary. First, explicit references to texts, theorists, movements, concepts, and events were pursued to map the implications of each statement and the strength of its allies in producing itself as truth. Connections were also made by mapping recurring terms such as 'human', 'rights', 'reality', and 'subject' across texts to explore their differential interpretations and applications. These connections helped to establish not only the limits of the discursive formation that gave occupational justice its sense and validity but also the parameters for sampling.

Ultimately, 33 discrete texts were sampled, ranging from short articles to entire books, though far more were read and analyzed to determine their relevance. Texts were chosen over interviews as the aim of the study was to explore whether published material that is widely accessible might support a form of political activism that is either unacknowledged in, or antithetical to, the stated aims of occupational justice theory.

In the case of sampling and recruiting human participants, procedures can be followed from other methodologies. However, special consideration of ethical issues should be made as critical research can involve oppressed, marginalized, vulnerable, and also already over-researched people. Time may need to be spent establishing relationships with communities so as to develop insight and an effective working relationship that does not simply extract data from the population and further disadvantage and disempower.

Data collection and analysis methods

The analysis methods best suited to critical theory are often preceded by the word critical. Critical discourse analysis (Fairclough, 2007), critical and postcritical ethnography (Noblit, Flores & Murillo, 2004), and critical hermeneutics or ideology critique (Vighi & Feldner, 2007) all signal their critical intentions. But participatory action research, case studies, narrative, historical, and sociological analyses can all be imbued with critical intent. When it comes to data collection and analysis in critical research, there is a lack of clearly defined rules or single method of best practice.

Critical research data comes in many forms including visual art, film, literature, performance, interview transcripts, policy, theoretical texts, architecture, conversation, observation, reflexive thought, music, and so on. The challenge for the critical theorist is matching data collection to the epistemological commitments of the project such that the data collected can answer the question posed. This means that the right data are collected from the right places, in the right way, and are flexible enough to change as the reflexive process dictates.

Analysis methods differ even more than potential data, as for each type of data, several methods could be used, but common to all methods is a very detailed attention to the position of the analyst and acceptance that the analyst is intimately related to the analysis.

I collected data iteratively in parallel with analysis. Each text was read at least twice to develop familiarity before analytically reading it to identify key statements (Foucault, 1969/2007), including verbal and written language, diagrams, and images, acts that functioned within and across texts to constitute a network of meaning. A table was produced for each text in which to record the key statements identified, their location in the text, as well as their connection to other statements within and across the text. In some cases, statements were as little as two words such as 'occupational potential', or as long as 100 words. Analysis took 18 months to complete including writing up the findings which was used as a reflexive strategy.

As stated in the previous section, texts were sampled based on their interconnections with other texts. Fairclough's (2007, p. 117) notion of "manifest intertextuality" structured this process as it fosters the pursuit of intertextual connections based on what a text presupposes, negates, narrates, or relies on for ironic effect. This approach was selected as it accorded with the explicitly stated epistemological commitments of the project including an operational definition of discourse, a specific theory of truth and power, and an exposition of how texts operate in concert with one another to produce truths within disciplines. When undertaking critical research it is recommended that such commitments be transparently reported and used to guide the selection of analysis tools. This ensures that tools are well suited to the data and the problem and provides rigor and validity to the research more broadly.

Findings from analysis were reported as a set of 12 propositions that were crucial to the coherence of occupational justice as a concept, but only apparent when viewing the network of connected statements. As emphasized earlier, findings are typically reported descriptively and include the data itself, how they were interpreted, and how connections were made. This informs the reader of the precise analytic steps undertaken but also defines key targets for social transformation by mapping those operations of truth and power that silently serve to oppress and subjugate. Where findings are reported thematically, it is crucial that each theme is supported descriptively so as to transparently demonstrate to the reader the process of each theme's production.

Rigor and ethics

> Critique is destruction as joy, the aggression of the creator.
>
> (Deleuze, 1962/2006, p. 87)

This quote provides a useful insight into the guiding principles of rigor and validity in critical research. The aim is not to accurately represent something but to change it. As such, validity is determined by how well the research has made possible something that was previously impossible (Rajchman, 1985), and rigor is ensured by deep and systematic reflexive practices. Critical theory is only interested in destroying present constructs to create new ones and is thus an "an agent that facilitates change" or catalyst (Brown, Stevenson & Trumble, 2002, p. 357). It is creative and purposeful, and the purpose is to disrupt the hegemonic status quo (Buchanan, 2010). Validity cannot therefore be determined by how well the research findings correspond to the phenomena of study (Lather, 1993). Instead critical theory determines validity by the extent to which the research has delivered those people it studied to new understandings of how their worlds are shaped such that they are better able to transform it (Kincheloe & McLaren, 2005).

Catalytic and transgressive validity

Catalytic validity refers to whether or not the research process has made possible something that was previously impossible. This might be a type of political action, the opportunity for voice or representation, or a new way of understanding a problem. The distinction between catalysis and causality is important. Causality would imply that the research unilaterally delivered transformative capacity, but as Marx said, critical theory is concerned with "self-clarification". While critical research aims to have an impact on reality the researcher must "consciously channel this impact so that respondents gain self-understanding and, ideally, self-determination through research participation" (Lather, 1986, p. 96). Catalytic validity is thus a collaborative creative project.

As with all creative projects, critical research will transgress disciplinary boundaries and cross the lines of existing taboos. It may reframe a problem, recommend a course of action, or implicate particular people and practices in ways that create discomfort and worry. This is because truly new creations do not conform to existing criteria of good or bad and thus force a transformation of what is considered good or bad.

Triangulation

Here the analyst is interrogating how the theoretical tools of the research are making the phenomenon visible and whether other ways of approaching the data might be of value. In terms of the mantis shrimp analogy used earlier, triangulation would involve using different cameras, maybe even a listening device or tactile input to understand the reef. In research terms it involves consulting alternative theories and methods or with experts from other disciplines to identify blind spots and presuppositions in the interpretation.

Construct validity – checking knowledge structures

In construct validity, the researcher asks whether the knowledge being constructed through the research process is accountable to the data. Has the researcher allowed the data to transform and change him or her, or has it simply been translated into existing knowledge structures without changing them? No matter how progressive, left or invested one is, such an approach is insufficiently reflexive. Construct validity involves being suspicious of the fact that your view of the reef and photograph of the reef look the same. The analyst must interrogate her own knowledge structures and how she is making the phenomena visible.

Face validity – checking with others

Face validity is designed to ensure that the knowledge constructed does not alienate the people it most powerfully affects. To what extent does it accord with their experience, language, and understanding? It means showing the photograph of the reef to the mantis shrimp that live there and working out how the picture differs from theirs. In research terms, it involves taking tentative findings to participants and refining them collaboratively. In the case of textual data, such as policies or literature, face validity is more difficult to achieve. Researchers must reflect on who is most affected by the texts and incorporate those views into their reflexive process. This might include those people targeted by the policy, regulated by the guidelines, or intended as a text's audience. Often times this reflexive process will generate data that is reported directly in publications.

Critiquing critical theory studies

This section synthesizes the discussion above into a discrete set of questions that can support examination of critical research (see Textbox 14.2).

Textbox 14.2   Critiquing critical theory studies – questions to ask

1   Can you see evidence that this paper accords in some way with the *seven themes* of critical research outlined in Textbox 14.1?
2   Does it use critical theory, or is it criticism espoused by someone with the 'correct political values'?
3   Does it *defend* an established position or *interrogate* one?
4   Does it *engage* with primary critical texts and issues of epistemology?
5   How could the findings *open new possibilities* for progress on the issue?
6   Is there evidence of *systematic reflexivity*?
7   Does it reduce the phenomena to '*social forces*'?
8   Does it engage with counterexamples and messy findings?

It is important to note that any attempt at a complete list would be misleading and dangerous. Many more questions could be asked as critical theory is by no means homogenous, and each critical tradition will have questions unique to its emphases.

Application to occupational science

Critical theory has a great deal to offer occupational science, and its increasing presence in the field has been widely heralded as timely and necessary (Laliberte Rudman, 2014; Whalley Hammell, 2011). It can furnish researchers with the capacity to undertake politically engaged research with the potential to transform society, the discipline, and the researcher. Critical research can provide insight into macroscale discursive forces that govern and regulate human occupation, shaping social organization and health outcomes. Furthermore, it still allows the discipline to critically reflect on its own assumptions and truth claims.

This latter focus is a particular interest of mine as it casts a critical lens back on ourselves to highlight the injustices that we ourselves perpetuate. This was especially so in my doctoral work which showed a profound irony with occupational justice. That is, to represent human rights politically, occupational science expounds a theory of human nature, natural law, and the distinction between science and politics. This means that, while occupational science does not uncritically generalize Northern metaphysics, enchantments, and beliefs to all people, it nonetheless claims to have discovered the "bedrock truths" (Seth, 2007, p. 190) that underpin these for all people. While all people have beliefs, we scientists alone have both beliefs AND the facts. I argue that tendering such facts to critique is a deeply discomforting experience, but this is precisely the ethical disposition required to support a different form of progress that might no longer be in our hands.

Application to occupational therapy

In relation to therapeutic practice several authors have challenged occupational therapists to reflect on unexamined presuppositions in theories of practice (Kinsella & Whiteford, 2009; Whalley Hammell, 2009). Kinsella and Whiteford (2009) have used the critical theory of Pierre Bourdieu to argue that practitioners must interrogate not only the validity of practice, but the conditions in which the knowledge that informs ideas of validity is produced. Whalley Hammell (2009) has drawn on feminist and postcolonial critical theories to clarify assumptions in what she describes as "Sacred texts" as a way of progressing occupational therapy beyond white middle class epistemologies. She has targeted unexamined notions of occupational categories (Whalley Hammell, 2009), spirituality, and the mind–body dualism (Whalley Hammell, 2011) in order to determine how knowledge can be produced in a manner that includes radically differing worldviews.

Another collective of practitioners has organized around the project of transgressing disciplinary, geographical, and political boundaries (Kronenberg, Simó Algado & Pollard, 2007; Kronenberg, Pollard, Sakellariou, 2011). Occupational therapists without borders have used various critical theories to understand how sociopolitical conditions affect the well-being of marginalized Southern communities in order to undertake explicitly political transformative practice. These practitioners contend that "politics is an aspect of human occupation and human relationships that can be found everywhere" (Kronenberg & Pollard, 2005, p.70). This small 'p' politics is not confined to formal places and processes of government but dispersed through the daily occupations of all people. Critical theory is used here to redefine health as a political issue and occupational therapy practice as an inescapably political intervention.

Reflection

Critical theory has deeply transformed my life by repeatedly unsettling my certainties. Relinquishing any sense of a timeless and fixed foundation for my values, behaviors, and ideas is an ongoing task that is both discomforting and hopeful. By the end of my doctoral work, I saw the Northern concept of nature as a significant barrier to occupational justice as it powerfully shapes the terms of political engagement and sustainable development. By turning my attention to questions of nature, ecological politics, and sustainable development I have been unsettled anew. Three provocateurs are significant.

1   Brassier (2007, p. xi) stated that "nature is not our or anyone's 'home', nor a particularly beneficent progenitor".
2   Morton (2010) told me that my ecological significance is akin to that of a B Grade celebrity in a slasher film in which no character is more important than the other and could die at any time.
3   Stengers (2002) claimed that not knowing what to do in the face of such challenges might provide the greatest hope for making significant progress.

Nonetheless, I still use critical theory to support research into the way that nonhumans act on humans, and what type of political representation nonhumans need in order to support sustainable development. The key learning from my experience with critical theory is that to critique anything, I must be vulnerable to critique myself.

Conclusion

Despite the wide-ranging remit of critical research and the histories of its emergence, I have stressed several key points in this chapter. First, critical research is an overt intervention in the phenomena of interest, not an activity that occurs around or about it. Second, critical research is not judgmental, as though one can sure footedly stand and denounce other people or positions. Critical research is a reflexive and uncertain process that can transform the footings of the researcher as much as the conditions being researched. Third, critical research must avoid reduction to readily available explanations that do nothing to open up new strategies for political action. Its purpose should be rich and intelligible descriptions of the conditions oppressing political actors (whether human or nonhuman) so that better futures can be imagined and actualized. Critical research is a proactive, transformative, and ethicopolitical research approach concerned with producing different worlds invested with hope.

References

Austin, J. (1975). *How to do things with words* (2nd ed.). Cambridge, MA: Harvard University Press.

Bennett, J. W. (2010). *Vibrant matter: A political ecology of things*. Durham, UK: Duke University Press.

Brassier, R. (2007). *Nihil unbound: Enlightenment and extinction*. New York: Palgrave Macmillan.

Brown, L., Stevenson, A., & Trumble, W. R. (Eds.). (2002). *Shorter Oxford English dictionary on historical principles* (5th ed.). Melbourne, Australia: Oxford University Press.

Brown, W. (2004). "The most we can hope for...": Human rights and the politics of fatalism. *The South Atlantic Quarterly, 103*(2/3), 451–463.

Bryant, L. (2011). The ontic principle: Outline of an object oriented ontology. In L. R. Bryant, N. Srnicek, & G. Harman (Eds.), *The speculative turn: Continental materialism and realism* (pp. 261–278). Melbourne, Australia: Re.press.

Buchanan, I. (2010). *Oxford dictionary of critical theory*. New York: Oxford University Press.

Butler, J. (1993). *Bodies that matter: On the discursive limits of "sex"*. New York: Routledge.

Butler, J. (2004). What is critique? An essay on Foucault's virtue. In S. Salih & J. Butler (Eds.), *The Judith Butler reader* (pp. 302–322). Malden, MA: Blackwell.

Butler, J. (2006). *Gender trouble: Feminism and the subversion of identity*. New York: Routledge.

Chiou, T. H., Kleinlogel, S., Cronin, T. W., Caldwell, R. L., Loeffler, B., . . . Marshall, J. (2008). Circular polarization vision in a stomatopod crustacean. *Current Biology, 18*(6), 429–434. doi:10.1016/j.cub.2008.02.066

Cronin, T. W., Caldwell, R. L., & Marshall, J. (2001). Tunable colour vision in mantis shrimp. *Nature, 411*(May), 547. doi:10.1038/35079184.

Cronin, T. W., & Marshall, N. J. (1989). A retina with at least ten spectral types of photoreceptors in a mantis shrimp. *Nature, 339*(May), 137–140.

Deleuze, G. (2006). *Nietzsche and philosophy* (H. Tomlinson, Trans.). New York: Columbia University Press. (Work originally published in 1962).

Fairclough, N. (2007). *Discourse and social change*. Cambridge, UK: Polity Press.

Foucault, M. (1977). *Discipline and punish: The birth of the prison* (A. Sheridan, Trans.). London, UK: Penguin. (Work originally published in 1975).

Foucault, M. (1978). *The history of sexuality 1: The will to knowledge* (R. Hurley, Trans.). London, UK: Penguin. (Work originally published in 1976).

Foucault, M. (1990). *The history of sexuality 3: The care of the self* (R. Hurley, Trans.). London, UK: Penguin. (Work originally published in 1984).

Foucault, M. (1992). *The history of sexuality 2: The use of pleasure* (R. Hurley, Trans.). London, UK: Penguin. (Work originally published in 1984).

Foucault, M. (1994). *The order of things: An archaeology of the human sciences*. New York: Random House. (Work originally published in 1963).

Foucault, M. (1997). What is critique? In S. Lotringer & L. Hochroth (Eds.), *The politics of truth* (pp. 23–82). Los Angeles, CA: Semiotexte.

Foucault, M. (2007). *The archaeology of knowledge* (A. Sheridan Smith, Trans.). London, UK: Routledge. (Work originally published in 1969).

Harman, G. (2011). *The quadruple object*. Alresford, UK: Zero Books.

Kincheloe, J. L., & McLaren, P. (2005). Rethinking critical theory and qualitative research. In N. K. Denzin & Y. Lincoln (Eds.), *The Sage handbook of qualitative research* (3rd ed., pp. 303–342). Thousand Oaks, CA: Sage.

Kincheloe, J. L., McLaren, P., & Steinberg, S. (2011). Critical pedagogy and qualitative research: Moving to the bricolage. In N. K. Denzin & Y. S. Lincoln (Eds.), *The SAGE handbook of qualitative research* (4th ed., pp. 163–178). Thousand Oaks, CA: Sage.

Kinsella, E., & Whiteford, G. (2009). Knowledge generation and utilisation in occupational therapy: Towards epistemic reflexivity. *Australian Occupational Therapy Journal, 56*(4), 249–258.

Kronenberg, F., & Pollard, N. (2005). Overcoming occupational apartheid: A preliminary exploration of the political nature of occupational therapy. In F. Kronenberg, S. Simó Algado, & N. Pollard (Eds.), *Occupational therapy without borders: Learning from the spirit of survivors* (pp. 58–86). Edinburgh, Scotland: Elsevier.

Kronenberg, F., Pollard, N., & Sakellariou, D. (Eds.). (2011). *Occupational therapies without borders volume 2: Towards an ecology of occupation-based practices.* Edinburgh, Scotland: Elsevier.

Kronenberg, F., Simó Algado, S., & Pollard, N. (2007). *Occupational therapy without borders: Learning from the spirit of survivors.* Edinburgh, Scotland: Elsevier.

Laliberte Rudman, D. (2005). Understanding political influences on occupational possibilities: An analysis of newspaper constructions of retirement. *Journal of Occupational Science, 12*(3), 149–160. doi:10.1080/14427591.2005.9686558.

Laliberte Rudman, D. (Online 2014). Embracing and enacting an 'occupational imagination': Occupational science as transformative. *Journal of Occupational Science.* doi:10.1080/14427591.2014.888970.

Lather, P. (1986). Issues of validity in openly ideological research: Between a rock and a soft place. *Interchange, 17*(4), 63–84.

Lather, P. (1993). Fertile obsessions: Validity after poststructuralism. *The Sociological Quarterly, 34*(4), 673–693.

Latour, B. (1988). Part II: Irreductions (A. Sheridan & J. Law, Trans.). *The pasteurization of France* (pp. 151–273). Cambridge, MA: Harvard University Press.

Latour, B. (2005). *Reassembling the social: An introduction to actor-network theory.* New York: Oxford University Press.

Latour, B., & Woolgar, S. (1986). *Laboratory life: The construction of scientific facts.* Princeton, New Jersey: Princeton University Press.

Mancuso, K., Hauswirth, W. W., Li, Q., Connor, T. B., Kuchenbeckler, J. A., . . . Neitz, M. (2009). Gene therapy for red-green colour blindness in adult primates. *Nature, 461*(7265), 784–787. doi:10.1038/nature08401.

Marx, K. (1888/1969). *Ludwig Feuerbach and the end of classical German philosophy* (W. Lough, Trans.). Moscow, USSR: Progress.

Marx, K. (1975). Letter to A. Ruge, September 1843 (R. Livingstone & G. Benton, Trans.). *Karl Marx: Early writings.* New York: Vintage.

Marx, K., & Engels, F. (1970), *The German ideology: Part one with selections from parts two and three, together with Marx's "Introduction to a Critique of Political Economy".* New York: International Publishers.

Morrow, R. A., & Brown, D. D. (1994). *Critical theory and methodology.* Thousand Oaks, CA: Sage.

Morton, T. (2010). *The ecological thought.* Cambridge, MA: Harvard University Press.

Noblit, G.W., Flores, S.Y., & Murillo, E.G. (2004). *Postcritical ethnography: An introduction.* Cambridge, UK: Cambridge University Press.

Patton, M. (2002). *Qualitative research and evaluation methods* (3rd ed.). Thousand Oaks, CA: Sage.

Rajchman, J. (1985). *Michel Foucault: The freedom of philosophy.* New York: Columbia University Press.

Sellar, B. (2012). Occupation and ideology. In G. Whiteford & C. Hocking (Eds.), *Critical perspectives on occupational science: Society, inclusion, participation* (pp. 86–99) Oxford, UK: Wiley.

Seth, S. (2007). *Subject lessons: The western education of colonial India.* Durham, UK: Duke University Press.

Stengers, I. (2002). A 'cosmo-politics' – risk, hope, change: A conversation with Isabelle Stengers. In M. Zournazi (Ed.), *Hope: New philosophies for change* (pp. 244–272). Annandale: Pluto Press.

Stepelevich, L. S. (2010). From Hegelian reason to Marxian revolution, 1831–48. In T. Nenon (Ed.), *The history of continental philosophy Volume I: Kant, Kantianism and idealism: The origins of continental philosophy* (pp. 237–263). Durham, UK: Acumen.

Vighi, F., & Feldner, H. (2007).Ideology critique or discourse analysis? *European Journal of Political Theory, 6*(2), 141–159. doi:10.1177/1474885107074347.

Whalley Hammell, K. (2009). Sacred texts: A sceptical exploration of the assumptions underpinning theories of occupation. *Canadian Journal of Occupational Therapy, 76*(1), 6–13.

Whalley Hammell, K. (2011). Resisting theoretical imperialism in the disciplines of occupational science and occupational therapy. *British Journal of Occupational Therapy, 74*(1), 27–33. doi:http://dx.doi.org/10.4276/030802211X12947686093602.

Zizek, S. (1994). *Mapping ideology.* London, UK: Verso.

Further reading

Foucault, M. (1997). *The politics of truth.* Los Angeles, CA: Semiotexte.

Latour, B. (2004). Why has critique run out of steam? *Critical Inquiry, 30*(2), 225–248.

Nenon, T. (2010). Immanuel Kant's turn to transcendental philosophy. In T. Nenon (Ed.), *The history of continental philosophy Volume I: Kant, Kantianism and idealism: The origins of continental philosophy* (pp. 15–47). Durham, UK: Acumen.

Rose, N. (1999). *Powers of freedom: Reframing political thought.* Cambridge, UK: Cambridge University Press.

15 Closing conversations

Shoba Nayar, Mandy Stanley, Eric Asaba,
Debbie Laliberte Rudman, Clare Wilding, and
Valerie Wright-St Clair

This book opened with a conversation, and now, as we come to a close, we offer this chapter, which is a transcript of part of a conversation that took place using Skype, between an international group of well established researchers who use qualitative methodologies. The purpose of the discussion was to invite these researchers, all of whom are contributing authors in this book, to share their thoughts regarding the strengths and challenges of engaging in qualitative research, and to offer some pearls of wisdom for undertaking qualitative research based on their experiences. Throughout the conversation, the researchers drew upon their chosen methodology to provide context to some of their comments. The conversation lasted for well over an hour, and as such, the transcript below has been edited; however we have sought to retain as much of the original dialog as possible. As a group we enjoyed engaging in this conversation and we trust, that in these final words, you will read something that resonates as you learn more about yourself as a qualitative researcher . . .

Shoba: What do you think are the strengths of qualitative research and the variances that exist within that term qualitative research?

Debbie: One of the places to start is what do we mean by qualitative research and what do we include in that term? It's so diverse that to try to get at the key of what makes it qualitative, I think is one of the challenges.

Mandy: I agree. Some years ago it seemed open ended questions at the end of a questionnaire were qualitative research and I'm pretty sure that's not the kind of qualitative research that we're talking about here. So what are the elements then, that holds or brings it together, into this thing we call qualitative research?

Valerie: One is the nature of the data, but I wonder whether it's where you're working inductively with the data that's gathered versus deductive. So maybe it's ways of working with data that is different than something where you are testing out some existing theory.

Eric: Maybe what we're also saying is that part of it is the method and another part is the methodology, and then another part of it is the techniques we use to look at text, non-numerical data is another way of saying it, and then the other part is how are we thinking about it. Maybe generating hypotheses could be one strength of this method; we don't know what we're going to test but we need to find out something is a nice way to begin.

Clare: I like that idea Val, especially that it's inductive rather than deductive. But with the non-numerical data it's interesting because I think sometimes you can actually start with some statistical data and start to explore patterns and ask questions that arise from the patterns that you see in the data. However, I do think it's that idea of not having a deduction or not having a hypothesis at the beginning that you're testing; rather trying to explore the world and understand what's happening in the observations that you make, in the data that you gather. And to me that's actually one of the strengths of qualitative research which is that it's about exploration and it's about not knowing, but the process of exploring and finding out.

Debbie: So, situated critically, in a critical paradigm, there's sometimes a struggle because I don't think of my work as inductive or deductive. It's something else, which doesn't necessarily have a word. Some people use abductive but for me there's that constant back and forth between the data and theory which I think happens in inductive approaches; but it's a misnomer to call critical work inductive because there are some ideas and values you bring to the data around power and oppression and issues of equity that you're looking for.

Mandy: And I was thinking before about not having any kind of preconceived ideas, but a lot of the time when you come to a study you do have some idea of what you might find. You know you're open to listening to people or looking to see what is there but often you've got some hunches already. That's the reality of it; and so you don't come completely free but for me, the beauty of qualitative research is in finding those things that are the taken-for-granted, and the unknowns that you reveal in the process. So even if you have a hunch, you still have to be open to what you find.

Debbie: I would say definitely I see that as a strength, that ability to question, unpack taken-for-granted, from various paradigms. So you're not starting with a preconceived notion of the way the world is, although you may be starting with a perspective that enables you to see some things and not other things and being very clear about what your perspective enables you to see and also knowing you won't see other things in your data because of that perspective. But you also have to push yourself beyond your perspective. For me, another strength is that qualitative allows a space for different kinds of voices to be articulated. So you're not starting with the researcher voice about the way the world is but engaging with varying kinds of multiple perspectives or multiple realities on the way the world is.

Valerie: And coming into that it feels one of the strengths is the sense of uncertainty in some ways; and I'm thinking particularly phenomenology there's that sense that you can work to try and get as close to possible to understanding something but there's an acceptance that you will never know it in its entirety and there needs to be a comfort with that but always perceive that there's something in the world that is worthy of more exploration and it's never going to be thrown into the light completely and we'll understand it from here on.

Shoba: For me it's about the human nature and that human voice. If I look at my work around migrants and refugees, policies and policy makers so easily box people into categories to deliver services or interventions or plan what we are going to do; and I think, for me, qualitative research brings the humanness back into it.

Clare: The power of stories; and for me that's one of the strengths of qualitative research. Stories are very compelling and they can really help us to understand a range of different perspectives and phenomena and situations through something that is quite simple but it really has a lot of resonance with people who are reading or engaging with the research.

Valerie: One of the other strengths around what we've been grouping here as qualitative research, is all of them call on the researcher(s) to declare or look at what the pre-understandings or the lenses are and put those out there and engage them in that process which isn't always done with things that we think of as being in the quantitative cluster. So I think understanding the lenses that you bring and pre-understanding is a strength of qualitative research. It's working with the otherwise taken-for-granted assumptions and the researcher becomes a part of that.

Debbie: I like the idea of power of story, and at multiple levels, because I am very interested in the power of the collected story which is another way to think about discourse. It's sort of a collective story that in a particular context comes to the fore either as a dominant story or a resisting story and I think story is something that helps us, maybe that's a branch across different types of approaches? Some are about that individual story and some are more collective stories. It seems a way to understand how people understand and act in the world is according to the stories they tell.

Eric: I agree and I think that one thing that challenges the sort of narrativity of it is, for instance, the video material where data might be qualitative, so to speak, and I'm thinking of some of the problems we have in our genre that have used that kind of data and made it narrative in a way but at first it's like not obviously narrative. But I'm in agreement, it's a strength of what we're calling qualitative I think.

Debbie: Another thing I like about qualitative, maybe it's a strength, is it's about relationships. It's about learning through relating to people. I think it's also a strength because that is how we learn about the world and learn about how to act in the world is through relationships and qualitative allows you to have relationships with people as a means to learn.

Clare: Yes people who participate in qualitative research, whether they're co-researchers or whether they're participants in a more traditional sense, there's an ability for them to learn a lot through that process of telling their own story and having a researcher witness that storytelling and reflect back to them and they can deepen their own understanding of their own stories and their own experiences. So I think that is a benefit of qualitative research.

Mandy: And I think that's why it has a real grab for occupational therapists and occupational scientists because building relationship and engaging in people's stories is part of what attracts us – maybe that's why we've gone into the profession or the discipline – so there's a natural fit for many people. Personally I don't mind doing quantitative stuff, but the numbers just seem cold, whereas the qualitative data, the stories, there's that richness there that's engaging and about relationship that I think nurtures both groups of people.

Eric: We're pointing at something which is storied in nature and that's quite important in terms of what we're doing in this kind of work.

Debbie: Right it's not just an open-ended response to something, it's imbued with some larger meaning related to this idea of story.

Eric: And it's not a decontextualized text, it's situated.

Valerie: Yes it's always situated in the world and I think that idea of text rather than narrative because other sorts of things are textual in nature but not necessarily spoken, but you kind of language them in the process of doing research. Text itself can be very diverse and has the potential to reveal the hidden or think or explore why things might be so at a deeper and reflective level or the what's going on or the how things are for people that doesn't become so visible when we're looking at patterns or numbers which have their own value and raise certain questions.

Clare: I think that what we're doing is telling conceptual stories so it doesn't really matter in what ways the data presents itself whether it's pictures or text or videos. It's understanding the world through creating a conceptual story that becomes something that we think about and that we feel and that we experience. Numbers in and of themselves have limited meaning but there is something in looking at, for example, population statistics and thinking about why is it that this particular group of people has this particular characteristic and why does that group of people have that particular characteristic, what is the difference there? So it's going beyond the numbers themselves. Qualitative researchers are less concerned about the raw numbers proving something but rather those numbers are a jumping off point to thinking about what's this underlying conceptual story that's going on here.

Shoba: Given the discussion thus far, the word that comes to my mind is complexity – the storied nature, the humanness, conceptualizing, the individual, community, population, it's complex. So what do you think then are some of the challenges or the tensions that we face when we undertake qualitative research?

Debbie: As someone who teaches qualitative methodologies, I think one of the tensions that already exists is how to teach it for those who are new to the subject, and how to teach in its own right without always doing the comparison to quantitative research.

Shoba: And Debbie do you find that same tension outside of the classroom in terms of when you are engaging in collaborations?

Debbie: Oh that's a leading question! It's a question of who one is collaborating with! Where one is submitting one's grant isn't it? Whether that's a tension you need to engage with or that's a tension you can work around. Knowing who your audience is or who you are working with, where you start that discussion I think varies.

Valerie: It feels again that some of this taken-for-grantedness in what is research and how we know things in the world comes from that assumed understanding, the enlightenment, that kind of scientific development has been so imbued within how we come to know the world that maybe that's why the researcher's assumptions have to be always revealed and shown because it's actually saying hey there may be other ways of trying to understand how it is in the world. So it feels like we need to poke it a little bit and shake it up but most people certainly within the Western society or nations have just come to think about how we gain knowledge through one particular way of understanding things.

Clare: It's a historical hangover that we can't really shake. You know there's always that comparison with quant and interestingly even within audiences that are sympathetic there can still sometimes be that tension that somehow what you're doing isn't quite right or legitimate and especially when we think about the kind of models that we adopt, for example, hierarchies of evidence, which just perpetuate those myths and misunderstandings.

Shoba: One of the motivations for doing this book is again, historically, I don't think we've been very good as occupational therapists or occupational scientists in really engaging in the complexity that is this thing called qualitative research. Each of you has brought the complexity through very clearly in your chapters, that understanding you can't just say you're doing critical discourse or phenomenology or photo voice without unpacking all the layers below to see what is this particular lens. However, I think often one of the tensions with qualitative research is the time required, not just the time for carrying out the study, but the time to really embrace and be the methodology.

Eric: I agree, besides the time consuming challenge it could be a strength in a way as well in that scaffolding is needed and I think that's what you're getting at right Shoba? It's very hard to pick up a chapter, read it and then go out and do it in a relevant way. It's often a process needed in order to get deep enough so that it's not just a description of something.

Valerie: I think we're saying it's many things but one of the tensions is for me to find publications where it's very evident that the whole project was informed by a particular lens or methodology or philosophy so that if one is wanting to gain a sense of, I'm not sure credibility is the right word, it's not a seeking that but I think it can be readily discredited when the particular approach or philosophy isn't really evident in many of the publications. Not to say it wasn't there in the research but it suggests it hasn't been when it's not showing in a publication.

Eric: And could part of the problem or challenge be in the structures in the venues in which we publish?

Debbie: To create a space to really show reflexivity in an article is really difficult. You can say you used these techniques end of sentence. And is there space to show it? And often there isn't it because of all the other things you need to put in there that the journal wants. It's very hard to find an article that shows the reflexivity, which I think is such an essential part of the process but it sort of gets washed out in the publication process.

Valerie: And one of the tensions then is what the reviewers look for, what journal editors look for and I think certainly the idea that someone might understand what it is you're aiming to do or why it is important to show certain ways of working through the research versus where reviewers might see that as quite superfluous. So a tension is perhaps the focus of the publications and maybe there aren't enough that allow for the sorts of things that you might judge the goodness of the research.

Mandy: I think that tension also comes through in working with ethics committees. I've had feedback on student work 'oh why aren't you doing a member check on the transcript' and questioning some of the procedures from a particular lens and we might be using a different one. I think it's all the time kind of battling that historical nature of qualitative research emerging in a serious way perhaps later than some of the more accepted approaches and it seems where people put in I'm going to do this particular statistic or analysis that people don't question that. There's much more questioning around the qualitative and perhaps not from an informed point of view.

Debbie: Yeah there seem to be particular words that you're supposed to use like member checks or saturation and if those words aren't there it can become problematic even if those words make no sense to the methodology you use, you know to claim saturation may be philosophically incompatible. I've certainly had that conversation with editors to say I can't use that word it doesn't fit and that can sometimes be a tension.

Eric: Or to get the question of how many will you include based on your power analysis?

Debbie: Yes. How do you know that's enough people?

Clare: I think it goes back to Shoba's idea that you know it does take time to embrace, what did you say, "embrace and be the methodology" – that's a nice way of saying it! People who are on ethics committees and reviewers and editors if they're not living that world already; it is difficult and it's a new language, a new culture that they then need to try and get their heads around and most of us don't have time to do that where we're pressured by many different activities to do.

Mandy: I want to go back to the comment that Shoba made about complexity because I think that's one of the strengths and you can explore complexity that's situated within people's lives, but it also brings lots of challenges and tensions including power and politics. So one of the things that I often feel challenged about is what right do I have as a researcher to take up people's time and to mine their minds and words for my benefit when they may not directly benefit from the research. And there usually is a power differential and I think we're much more cognizant of that as qualitative researchers than quantitative, although maybe my more quantitative colleagues would argue with me on that one!

Debbie: Yeah it's that sort of are we doing research on, with or for, and how you position yourself in relationship to those issues, because I think qualitative research can do any of those. It can be on something, it can be for something, or it can be with. And how you position yourself in relationship to that I think is very important and to think of not treating your participants as sort of data but thinking about the kind of dignity that exists in your research and the relationships that you build. But yes sometimes feeling that you're stripping people of their experiences and thinking about the broader question of why are you doing that?

Clare: Recently I've been at the other end, producing of a report that is hundreds of pages long, and I just think very, very few people are going to read that. They'll read the executive summary which is four pages long and they'll ignore a lot of the complexity and richness that went into the creation of that report and that understanding. Again I think that it's a strength to have that complexity and to capture it and if you really go into it you can get a good understanding of a situation but on the flip side there is that complexity that can work against you because people just don't want to engage with it or don't have the time to engage with it.

Valerie: I think there's another perspective and that's for what ends or purpose? And when money is tight and bodies are funding research they want outcomes and answers and directions for how services should be funded. So I think one of the tensions is fitting in with the whole funding structure and forces that tie those whole complex social problems, particularly when there isn't an outcome that is predictive in nature. And where the time of the researcher is not funded, and qualitative methodologies philosophically call for a lot of engaging over time with data, one of the tensions is you bring a lot of yourself and commitment to the outcomes without necessarily being well funded to do the research.

Clare: Yeah, in some ways qualitative research is inexpensive in that it doesn't require a lot of specialized equipment or labs or computing, but the expense is a personal cost for the researcher in terms of time and commitment. I think when you engage in a qualitative research project you live with it, you live it yourself as a researcher for a period of time, it gets under your skin and that can be a hidden cost or experience that we don't often talk about.

Debbie: And for me that's the transformational potential. That it's not just transforming understandings but that you as a researcher transform through the research and the project so that I can say what I understood about aging when I started doing qualitative research in aging, my understanding has been transformed many times through engagement in many different kinds of projects and for me that's a strength but it's also a challenge because your voice changes and your understanding changes through time and you can look at earlier work and say I think I missed something in that, I understand now.

Valerie: And I think Clare's and Eric's point before that that the participants engaging in the process perhaps because of the reflective or exploratory reflected nature of it is that they can also be transformed in their own ways of making sense of things or how they understand things in their own world so, it's a tension and strength and it's not one or the other but it offers benefits as well.

Shoba: Given the complexities and the tensions that we've talked about, what advice would you give to occupational therapists/scientists starting out on a research career using qualitative approaches?

Eric: I think for me a really valuable way to start was to find somebody who was really good at doing qualitative research and be scaffolded into a thinking and a group and a dialogue and a context in which to make mistakes and to learn parallel to doing the more traditional scholarly sort of read and do. For me that was really helpful and that's why I would probably give that recommendation to somebody else as well.

Mandy: I agree. I have heard the term minus mentoring; I think sometimes you can attach yourself to people who actually don't do things very well and so you can learn lots of wrong ways. So it's finding somebody who does really good qualitative work and working with them. There are some things that you can't get from reading, you know you do need to read but I don't think I'm the only person who is an experiential learner. One of the examples that I can think of is when you get to the analysis and you're kind of the first full pass over the analysis and you think okay yes I've got it, I've got my themes, or I've got my categories, but then when that experienced person says to you okay that's descriptive now you've got to lift it into something more conceptual – how do I do that you know? It's hard getting that.

Shoba: Okay, imagine I am a beginner, where do I find someone who is experienced or well versed in this work?

Val: It's not just a good qualitative researcher; it's many things. To me you need someone who is very steeped in that way of thinking and doing and being in the world and doing research because it's that philosophical methodological integrity that feels like you need the guidance on as a novice researcher always has that integrity.

Debbie: When I think about the colleagues that I connect with to work with, that's often based on reading their work and it somehow speaks to me. I read what they've written and I think you know this resonates, I can see a connection point here, I could see how I could have a critical discussion with this person, how they write, what they write. That's always important before I embark on a potential collaboration with someone is to read something they've written and to see if I can see something of myself in conversation with that.

Eric: To me there's no way to know whether it's good or not. I wouldn't want to be the one that says that is good or not good but rather there are many ways to do it and so I think that once one takes the step that says okay well this person seems to be doing a lot of stuff, they're in a setting where there seems to be support for this I'm going to try it out. I think it's quite important to learn, to learn that once, and then to be creative after that to challenge it, as opposed to sort of doing it half heartedly and then trying something else half heartedly because then it's hard to know where it is that one's challenging something.

Debbie: The other thing that I always tell students or things we always have discussions about is patience and trust. It is a long complex process to engaging in any kind of qualitative research and methodology and to have that patience it will take time for the question to formulate, it will take time for the analysis to coalesce and we're in a world that wants us to do things according to specific time lines and sometimes you need to just wait, wait for a bit and to trust things like your engagement with the data and to trust that although one moment you feel utterly confused, another moment you might just have a great insight and I think that it's that non-linearity and that iterative process to trust it.

Mandy: Yeah I was thinking iterative process as you were talking because that applies not just to the data collection and the analysis but also in the writing and in many ways you haven't even quite finished the analysis until you're writing it up because you're still sorting it out in your head, what is the best way to present this that honors the participants and it makes sense and is cohesive, and that takes a number of goes. The thing that I would like to add to patience and trust is humility. I don't think you can be a good qualitative researcher without approaching it with humility and that it's actually not about you as a researcher but about the participants and their stories.

Clare: I agree with all of the things that have been said so far. With the time stuff, I say that that it's a bit like building a house, you need to make a time budget then double it! It always takes longer and costs more than you think it's going to. Also, it's great to work with someone who's talented and you connect with, but that's not always possible, but I still think that it's better to work, especially as a novice, to work with others rather than in isolation. Sometimes I see students who are reluctant to share their ideas or to talk over their data and I think that's a problem for them because it doesn't really allow them to have their ideas challenged or to think in other ways and it's really good to speak about it with someone else and it's much more fun.

Mandy: Yeah I think many of us formed study groups when we were doing our PhDs or when we started doing qualitative research. I did grounded theory for my PhD and I really bonded with some others because they were also using the same approach and we would get together and look at each other's data and talk about it. So you're using that reflexivity and peer debriefing to help understand it better and work through it and I would really encourage people to do that.

Clare: And there can also be surprising sources of inspiration and information. I remember when I was doing my masters and grappling with phenomenology and Heidegger. I read a cartoon book called *Heidegger for Beginners* and it was the first time I understood what it was all about, I had no idea before then! That then gave me an entry into the other more complicated texts but I needed to get that really basic kind of understanding first, so you know people might laugh when you say you've read a cartoon book about philosophy but it was helpful.

Eric: Another thing that I thought really meaningful with regard to learning qualitative research of different sorts, was I had one sort of method that I was getting into as a PhD student and then I came to a different context as a postdoc and I met people who were using the same term but in a different way. And so I was challenged to think about the kind of methods I had been using and then started to work with people who were using other things like phenomenology and that was a new world. I was keen on interpreting things and I was being told to bracket my biases and so then it opened up this dialogue right, well what do you mean by that? How do I do that? And try to understand how somebody else is looking at this. So for every step we take, to sort of develop a richness of how we're using a particular approach, if we make a conscious effort to step out of our comfort zone and step into somebody else's comfort zone, I think we will sort of get into some sort of debate around well what do you mean? I think as long as it can be a healthy debate it's quite useful. I've enjoyed it personally and maybe not all people can be in that environment but if you have the possibility for me that's been a really interesting thing to do that.

Valerie: One of the things I would give advice on is the thinking through why you're doing it a certain way and what guides that. It's not thinking there is one way but you've got a reason why you chose this methodology or why you work with the data in this way so I think it's understanding some of those reasons, what's guiding how you're working or how you're thinking about things. Maybe one of the other bits, certainly for interpretive phenomenology is to be comfortable with uncertainty and knowing that you're actually not going to know. You might get closer to understanding but I think that was maybe what Mandy was saying with humility, not just coming into it but going out where you end up is not the definitive point. So having a comfort in engaging in the thinking and writing. If you don't like engaging in writing it's not a good methodology for someone to use! So it's kind of knowing who you are and what you might bring to a project that also is part of what's important. That sense that yes you can engage in a way of thinking or questioning that just feels right. I don't say that you don't always step outside your comfort zone, but sometimes the fit just isn't there and knowing yourself as a person it's actually important as a researcher stepping somewhere in the field.

Debbie: Yes I agree with that because I think if any of us reflect on where we started and where we are now, personally it took me a long time to find my comfort, explore different kinds of methodologies and paradigms and I feel pretty comfortable where I am now but now I'm beginning to read new stuff that's sort of putting some holes in that and thinking okay how do I keep moving. So that notion there isn't a static place to be as a qualitative researcher and cautioning students about that like where you are now may not be where you are at the end of your project, it may not be where you are 10 years from now and it may be but that openness to thinking otherwise I think is really crucial in your development as a qualitative researcher.

Clare: I've really enjoyed that about qualitative research Debbie. I love the creativity of it and even the blending of different types of methods. It just allows you to take tangents that you wouldn't otherwise have thought about and it allows you to uncover information or discover information that you wouldn't have otherwise had access to.

Debbie: Yeah so I think that license to be creative and thinking about creativity as part of the process and how you bring creativity into this thing called science or research.

Mandy: So it requires a lot of cognitive flexibility and that ability to sit with the messiness and the incongruity for awhile. If you're somebody that likes things all neat and tidy and boxed up, then engaging in some of the analysis particularly would probably be troubling and you've got to trust! It's also about the thinking and that when you're working with the data it has to take time and you have to sit with the not knowing for quite a while and keep working at it to come out with some findings. Some people when they're starting think oh I'm not doing this right or I'm obviously not good at this but it actually is hard and you can't force it, you have to keep at it but you will get there, so trusting, but sitting with the messiness for a bit longer will get there in the end.

Clare: Good point! You really have to trust the process and step into that void of not knowing and know that you don't know and just hang around there for a while until one day it does fall into place. I've told that to students and it's quite funny watching them grapple and try and force it to happen and then you know they change their ideas, they go through so many different things and then one day it does kind of fall into place.

We wish you well as you find your 'place' in the world of qualitative research!
Shoba and Mandy

Index

.

Printed in the United States
by Baker & Taylor Publisher Services

Printed in the United States
by Baker & Taylor Publisher Services